THE FIRST YEAR®

HIV

An Essential Guide for the Newly Diagnosed

BRETT GRODECK is a longtime AIDS activist and accomplished writer. HIV-positive since 1987, his articles have appeared in *Chicago* magazine, the *Chicago Reader,* and *Men's Fitness* magazine. He's written and edited for various medical publications and held positions with Edelman Public Relations, RAND Corporation, and Symantec Corporation. As a patient advocate, he is a consultant for the Food and Drug Administration. Grodeck lives in Los Angeles, California.

THE COMPLETE FIRST YEAR® SERIES

The First Year—Age-Related Macular Degeneration by Daniel L. Roberts
The First Year—Cirrhosis by James L. Dickerson
The First Year—Crohn's Disease and Ulcerative Colitis by Jill Sklar
The First Year—Fibroids by Johanna Skilling
The First Year—Fibromyalgia by Claudia Craig Marek
The First Year—Hepatitis B by William Finley Green
The First Year—Hepatitis C by Cara Bruce and Lisa Montanarelli
The First Year—HIV by Brett Grodeck
The First Year—Hypothyroidism by Maureen Pratt
The First Year—IBS by Heather Van Vorous
The First Year—Lupus by Nancy Hangar
The First Year—Multiple Sclerosis by Margaret Blackstone
The First Year—Parkinson's Disease by Jackie Hunt Christensen
The First Year—Prostate Cancer by Christopher Lukas
The First Year—Rheumatoid Arthritis by M.E.A. McNeil
The First Year—Scleroderma by Karen Gottesman
The First Year—Type 2 Diabetes by Gretchen Becker

THE FIRST YEAR®

HIV

An Essential Guide for the Newly Diagnosed

Second Edition, Completely
Revised and Updated

Brett Grodeck

Foreword by Daniel S. Berger, M.D.

MARLOWE & COMPANY ■ NEW YORK

THE FIRST YEAR®—HIV
Second Edition: An Essential Guide for the Newly Diagnosed

Copyright © 2003, 2007 by Brett Grodeck
Foreword copyright © 2007 by Daniel S. Berger, M.D.
Copyright © 2003 by Tanya Maiboroda for illustrations
appearing on pages 44, 45 and 112

Published by
Marlowe & Company
An Imprint of Avalon Publishing Group, Incorporated
161 William Street, 16th Floor
New York, NY 10038

AVALON
publishing group incorporated

The First Year® and A Patient-Expert Walks You Through
Everything You Need to Learn and Do® are trademarks of
the Avalon Publishing Group, Inc.

Library of Congress has cataloged the previous edition as follows:
Grodeck, Brett.
    The first year—HIV : an essential guide for the newly
diagnosed / by Brett Grodeck.
        p. cm.
Includes bibliographical references and index.
    ISBN 1-56924-490-1
    1. HIV infections—Popular works. I. Title: HIV.
II. Title.
RC606.64.G765 2003
362.1'969792—dc21   2003041270

This edition:
ISBN-10: 1-60094-013-7
ISBN-13: 978-1-60094-013-2

10 9 8 7 6 5 4 3 2 1

Designed by Pauline Neuwirth,
    Neuwirth and Associates, Inc.

Printed in the United States of America

Contents

CONTENTS

Foreword

By Daniel S. Berger, M.D.

THE HIV epidemic serves as a decisive model for what the power of human spirit can endure and accomplish. There have always been complex issues surrounding AIDS. Even now, there isn't a day that passes without the deep impressions made by the struggles of those early years of AIDS. While we have suffered many losses, we are obliged to recognize the achievements and progress made during a relatively short time of this history.

Some of the credit is owed to AIDS activism. Back in the day, it was the AIDS activists who brought necessary public attention to HIV. It was the AIDS activists who had been instrumental in altering government policy to approve medications through fast-track programs, helping ensure greater survival for those with HIV. With the help of AIDS activism, other life-threatening diseases have been able to take advantage of this fast-track approval process as well. AIDS advocacy and politics continue to interface. Overall, individuals with the virus are able to enjoy a much brighter outlook.

Determination and commitment contribute to reaching a better "sense of well-being" and health in HIV infection. Factors, once considered as outside the mainstream, including nutrition and lifestyle issues, are understood to be important and crucial in concert with scientifically based antiviral treatment. Even if you're not at the point of needing to explore antiviral treatments, inevitably you will be faced with HIV-related health issues. This book contains important information you need to make critical decisions.

Being HIV-positive poses many unique challenges. The hallmark of HIV infection is its damage to the immune system. Without proper treatment, various unusual infections (known as opportunistic infections), which ordinarily do not cause disease in normal individuals, have a greater propensity to develop. HIV invades other parts of the body and, depending on the specific organ systems that are affected, other symptoms can occur. But the good news is that that nearly every HIV-impacted individual can be empowered to control the disease and improve his or her health. We have gained much knowledge regarding the many facets of controlling HIV. The quality-of-life has vastly improved for those with the virus. Today individuals can avoid or overcome the historically pervasive problems of AIDS during the 1980s and early 1990s. In fact, there is little precedence for a disease to have begun with so much tragedy and hopelessness and to have evolved so quickly into a chronic manageable disease.

The mainstay of HIV treatment uses antiviral drugs from three main classes. Known as the "treatment cocktail," this combination of three (or sometimes four medications) from the classes of nucleosides, non-nucleosides, and protease inhibitors together halt HIV replication from inside human cells. But remarkably, therapy for HIV disease continues to be an ever-changing dynamic. Advances continue in finding new ways to attack the virus. One new line of attack employs a novel antiviral class of *integrase inhibitors*. While already making a huge impact for patients failing HIV treatments, integrase inhibitors are also being studied as initial drug cocktails for persons recently diagnosed. Another relatively new drug class, called entry and fusion inhibitors, block the binding of the virus to the CD4 T-cell. This class of drugs continues to be applied for patients who may fail therapy later.

Other advances include novel protease inhibitors, effective against highly resistant HIV. Solid accomplishments have occurred in reducing the number of pills needed per drug cocktail and decreasing the frequency of dosing. These continue to improve with each passing year. We have witnessed the arrival of the first triple-drug combination (a total regimen) in one pill taken only once daily. As HIV treatment progresses, it is likely that you will be taking more and more patient-friendly drugs that come in fewer and fewer numbers of pills.

Nutrition has always been a primary concern of HIV disease. Years ago, wasting was a common problem. Today, however, body-shape changes are a pressing complication. These changes are caused by fat redistribution, often coinciding with elevated levels of cholesterol and triglycerides. While the recent advance of a growth-hormone releasing factor has shown promise in treating this condition, there are still other emerging challenges, including diabetes and cardiovascular disease as patients grow older.

As a physician I stress the importance of remaining steadfast and stubborn with health maintenance. HIV infection should not become a distraction against planning for a long, healthy future. The tools of nutrition, physical fitness, and stress reduction are important with simplifying one's life; each are keys to successfully managing HIV. I am proud to be part of a book that places a large emphasis on these values. Brett Grodeck offers much practical guidance combined with easy-to-read introductions on scientific issues. He will help you understand the deadly consequences of using crystal meth, which has been a burgeoning problem within the HIV community. Brett also provides valuable advice to help you avoid contracting other infections, such as hepatitis B and C, herpes, and HPV. These can complicate your health. A dedicated chapter is also devoted to the importance of counseling and support in managing stress and depression; both can occur at any time during the life of someone with HIV. The friendly language—peppered with humor—makes *The First Year–HIV* enjoyable reading while also empowering, providing many adjunctive strategies for thriving with HIV.

I have known Brett for many years. He was involved in starting the first magazine for HIV-positive individuals. Subsequently, he became editor of the HIV treatment journal called *Positively Aware* in Chicago. He helped develop the journal into a prominent, nationally respected magazine. Today it remains among the finest available tools to educate HIV-positive individuals. Brett and I have engaged in frequent in-depth conversations, spanning various HIV-related subjects, and he often showed a knack for understanding and coming up with fresh perspectives from an HIV-positive point of view. Revising this edition of *The First Year–HIV,* Brett carefully updated the book with the latest emerging topics and, once again, manages to inject his unique personal insight.

The experience of reading this book will prove to you that there is more to treatment than medications, antiviral drugs, and doctor visits. The detailed approach of this book covers a broad variety of issues, drawn from many successful patients, experienced physicians, and thought leaders in the field of HIV. It is truly our intent that this book inspire you to continue living a long, healthy, and productive life.

DANIEL S. BERGER, M.D., is a clinical assistant professor of Medicine at the University of Illinois at Chicago and is founder and medical director of Chicago's largest private HIV treatment and research center, Northstar Healthcare. Dr. Berger has conducted more than one hundred clinical research trials in HIV therapeutics. He serves on the board of directors for the AIDS Foundation of Chicago and is a consultant and regularly featured columnist of *Positively Aware*. His column "The Buzz" is a well known fixture and routinely featured on TheBody.com Web site. Dr. Berger also serves on the HIV Medical Issues Committee for the Illinois AIDS Drug Assistance Program. Dr. Berger was the 2006 recipient of the Charles E. Clifton Leadership Award of Test Positive Aware Network in Chicago.

Preface to the Second Edition

WITH EVERY passing year, HIV medicine improves. Today, the gold-standard medicine for HIV is one pill that's taken once a day. The side effects are minimal and the benefits more than compensate for the alternative. I've made every attempt to incorporate the latest information on HIV medicine and treatment in this second edition of *The First Year—HIV*.

These days, however, the biggest problem is not the virus; unfortunately, it's people. The virus can be treated. But there are no pills for the people in your life who may react to you with fear or ignorance. In general, society continues to hold on to its irrational fears. In the United States, HIV and related stigma is rampant. When you test positive for HIV, suddenly you become the direct target of these irrational fears.

At the end of the day, HIV is transmitted by drugs or sex. Like it or not, that's our common denominator. And that's what I've emphasized in this edition of the book. Over the years, the shame can eat away at your self esteem, making you and your health vulnerable in other ways. In this new edition, I've emphasized a few areas of vulnerability that can be a concern for many people who are newly diagnosed with HIV. I also offer ways to cope with specific incidents of stigma, lifestyle issues, as well as ways to keep yourself as healthy as possible.

Introduction

I WAS lost when I first moved to Los Angeles. At first, the roads in L.A. didn't make sense to me. I'm from the Midwest and highways there usually radiate from a downtown area to the suburbs. In L.A., the term is *freeways,* and they connect Sacramento, Palm Springs, and San Diego. When I arrived in L.A., I knew that road signs to San Diego meant *south,* Sacramento meant *north,* and Palms Springs meant *east.* That was fine, except there were no signs pointing me to the local Wal-Mart and back.

Soon enough, my friend Nancy gave me a book. Actually, it was a large map, but in the form of a book. It laid out the roads and freeways of L.A. and I stashed the guide in my car. It helped somewhat. But it wasn't until Nancy began offering her experience and advice that I became at ease with driving in L.A. Now, I know to stay off the San Diego Freeway during rush hours. I remember to avoid the freeways near Dodger stadium and the Staples Center before a Dodgers or Lakers game. And I can now find my way to several different Wal-Marts—and get back home.

You might feel lost when you first discover you have HIV. I know when I discovered I was HIV-positive in 1987, I felt lost too. And it was far worse than I felt when I moved to L.A. Hearing the HIV-positive news yourself might transform your once-familiar world into a foreign place. You might be wondering: How do I find a doctor? What should I do next? Whom do I tell?

Well, there are no easy answers. HIV is a complicated condition. But there are many common things that people with HIV confront over time. In some ways, this book is a little like a roadmap of those issues. One difference, however, is that this book also offers the human element, the experiences, and the wisdom of others who have been in the same boat. Taken together, the two perspectives can help guide you toward more-informed and better decisions today and in the years to come.

What happened to me

I didn't have any noticeable symptoms when I tested positive for HIV at the age of twenty-one. I took an HIV test because I thought it was the right thing to do. I was shocked when I discovered that it was positive. For many years, the hardest part of having HIV was just knowing that I had it.

For the first few years, my immune system held steady. I didn't need HIV medications. But that eventually changed. Slowly over time, my immune system began to lose the battle it was fighting. As my immune system lost ground, minor symptoms developed, like swollen lymph nodes and skin problems. I felt tired a lot. Over time, I experienced a few more symptoms. I got some irritating warts on my feet; cold sores in the corners of my mouth; inexplicable bruises here and there; and my tongue sometimes burned when I ate spicy foods.

My response to my declining health was to keep closer tabs on the latest medical research. I kept very informed. However, I also knew that surviving wasn't just about gathering information. A *New England Journal of Medicine* article doesn't usually say much about how to discuss HIV with friends and family.

I figured one way to navigate through the emotional and social aspects of having HIV was by talking with other people. Eventually, I met other people who were also HIV-positive and became close friends with many of them. I learned new ways of thinking about situations I thought were hopeless. Sometimes, I learned valuable details from friendly, informal conversations with other people.

It's not uncommon to live with HIV for over twenty years like I have. I plan on living to at least the age of retirement. In the early years of my HIV, I wasn't as optimistic. In fact, I never wore a seat belt in a car back then. "Why bother?" I thought. Now that I'm healthy, I'm far more worried about getting in a car accident on the Los Angeles freeways than I am about getting sick from HIV.

How to use this book

Unlike a map, this book considers the human element. The chapters are laid out in a way that breaks down the big picture. I have parsed out small, bite-size portions of information that you can absorb right away. The small portions are arranged according to what is most relevant to most people right off the bat. Sometimes I outline the essentials of a complicated topic—like HIV medicine—in an early chapter, and then discuss it later in more detail. The book then moves on to the more subtle aspects of dealing with HIV.

It's great if you got this book on the first day after testing positive for HIV, but it's hardly necessary. If you've had HIV for years, you might be tempted to skip forward. That's fine, but some chapters are like scaffolding around a building. The top part of the scaffolding depends on the foundation at the bottom.

There will be days, perhaps even months, when you'll need a break from thinking about HIV. You might only be able to deal with reading Day 1 through Day 7 right now, and that's fine. You can always come back to the book a month down the road, when your mind has adjusted. Newly diagnosed or not, I encourage you to start from the beginning and work through the information at your own pace. In some cases, however, your current situation might require you to jump forward to a specific chapter.

Each Day, Week, or Month chapter is divided into a Living and a Learning section. The Living sections focus on the intangible stuff, like emotions, common concerns, or philosophies that doctors use when prescribing HIV medicine. The Learning sections generally focus on a few concrete things you can do—or shouldn't do—to help you stay healthy (such as quitting smoking, improving your diet, or getting more exercise). The choice is always yours, but at least you'll know your options.

Some terms in the book will show up in **boldface**. This means these words are defined in more detail within the glossary located at the back of this book. You'll also find a few signposts throughout the book. They designate the end of the first seven days, the first month, and first six months. When you reach these milestones, stop and pat yourself on the back, because absorbing this stuff isn't easy.

I will not prescribe

I am not a doctor. I will not prescribe for you. That decision is best left to you and your doctor or healthcare provider. Furthermore, HIV medicine changes quickly over time. Every year, new blood tests, drugs, drug combinations, and side effects will continue to emerge. What's right for you today may not be right for you five years from now. I only hope to provide a collection of general principles that have stood the test of time and personal experiences that have helped other people with HIV before you.

Where the focus is

I have focused on things that are relevant to most people who are newly diagnosed with HIV. Of course, if you've had the virus for a longer time, this book is still very useful. It covers a wide range of issues and offers suggestions for anyone affected by HIV.

I have steered clear of the unnecessary details about HIV medicine. Individual drugs and strategies come and go. For example, doctors at one time thought the best approach was to offer HIV medicine to all people early in HIV disease. This "hit hard, hit early" approach has fallen out of favor today, and has been replaced with a "hit hard, but wait longer" approach. New drugs and new tests may alter things again in the future.

I think it's important for you to know a few things about me and this book. In the past, when I wrote articles for HIV treatment publications, they were often funded by the pharmaceutical companies. Sometimes this fact influenced the information I wrote. I want you to know that this book is entirely funded and produced by my publisher, Marlowe & Company. I have no connection with pharmaceutical companies, either financially or otherwise. I think it's important for you to know that. I also think it's important for you to be on the lookout for possible pharmaceutical company involvement in anything you read about HIV.

Keep on learning

Thanks to a road map and advice from friends, I've learned how to find my way through Los Angeles. In the same way, this book will help you better navigate through the complexities of living with HIV.

People are different and they absorb information in different ways. Some people learn best by listening to or talking with another person. This book will help you locate those who can help you, especially with things like health care. Other people absorb information through the written word or the Internet. This book offers ways to assess the quality of the information you may encounter.

Some people may slam the door on information related to HIV. They more or less may choose not to think about the virus at all. Sometimes, a dose of denial is perfectly understandable (certainly, I went through periods of denial). But understand that there are certain times in HIV disease when denial carries a higher price. If you pay attention to your health now, you might save yourself some headaches in the future. You might have more peace of mind. This book will help you understand what choices and options you may encounter down the road.

You Can Manage HIV

RELAX, HIV is a completely different condition than it was a few years ago. Today, things are better. An HIV-positive diagnosis does not mean an inevitable decline in health, as it once did. In fact, the future is bright for people who are newly diagnosed with the virus—and things get better with every passing year.

If you haven't kept up on all the latest progress in HIV and medicine, your positive diagnosis may be quite upsetting. What you've learned about the virus has probably come from newspapers or television. Images of sickly people and hospital beds may be floating around your mind. Those images, however, speak of the old days, before 1996. That's when HIV medicine turned the corner and got dramatically better. And the outlook for people with the virus continues to improve.

You might know a little about HIV or AIDS. Perhaps you even know someone who is HIV-positive. If you're somewhat knowledgeable about the virus, you might be less concerned about your future. Instead, your worries may be focused on other people in your life, people close to you, those who may be less informed than you are. How partners, spouses, family members, or friends will respond to the news may be a bigger cause of worry for you. For now, it's a good idea to focus on you and taking care of yourself.

Testing HIV-positive can be scary. People respond to the news in different ways. Whatever your beliefs about the virus may be, the bottom line is this: Today's outlook for people with HIV is very optimistic. "People with HIV can have a full life and live a normal life expectancy if they do the right things," says Daniel S. Berger, M.D., a physician who has been treating people with HIV for many years.

This book is all about "doing the right things." But what's right for one person can be wrong for another. To make it all more complicated, what's right today may not be right tomorrow. Medicine changes over time. However, the basic rules, general guidelines, and the experiences of many people before you will always hold true over time. This is what you'll find in this book.

Having HIV means many things

Having HIV does not mean you have AIDS. A positive HIV test result only means that you have been infected with the virus. Having HIV does not mean that you will feel the effects of the virus immediately, nor does it mean that you have AIDS. Without intervening HIV medicine, the average time between initial infection and the development of the symptoms associated with AIDS is about ten years.

You might not need HIV medicine for many years. Depending when you were infected with the virus and how your immune system has responded to it, you may not need medicine anytime soon, perhaps not for years. Some people live for fifteen or twenty years without medicine. However, the only way to be sure is to see a doctor and have special blood tests performed. These blood tests can tell you much about the strength of your immune system.

HIV medicine is good now and it's getting better every year. The good news about HIV is not just about the medicine, which, incidentally, is effective and safe when used correctly. The untold story is about all the different blood tests that are available now to help guide your medical decisions. Years ago, doctors made educated guesses about how to fight the virus. Today, new blood tests can describe with precision what kind of HIV is in your body and how well HIV medicine will work for you. Both the drugs and the tests are great reasons for optimism.

You can continue to have an active and full life. Having HIV should not stop you from pursuing the life you wanted before your diagnosis. There are no medical reasons why you can't be just as active as you were before. This includes pursuing athletic goals, traveling to foreign countries, earning a college degree, or achieving success in your job or career. Furthermore, there are no medical reasons why you can't have a traditional family, find a spouse or a partner, or pursue sexual relationships with other people.

You've already taken one of the hardest steps: You had the courage to take an HIV test. This means you've learned the truth about what's happening to you. Now, you're reading this book to learn even more. You are taking control of your health and not letting your health control you.

It's true that things may be tough for you in the next year. The days, weeks, and months ahead may feel like a roller coaster of fears, emotions, and unfamiliar experiences. But understand that you're not alone. Many people have gone through similar experiences. The purpose of this book is to describe the lessons learned from these people before you. These lessons can help you today and in the days to come.

Whatever your initial response was to testing HIV-positive, remember that you have more control than you might think. It's easy to forget. You might choose to jump in and learn everything you can about the virus. You might choose to take a vacation from HIV for a time, knowing you'll deal with things later. Or you might just pretend you never tested HIV-positive in the first place. It's always your call. It's up to you to decide what course you want your life—and your HIV—to take.

IN A SENTENCE:

> *By finding out your HIV status, you're already taking control of your health.*

Your New Identity as a Person with HIV

WHEN I think about myself, I see myself as male, Caucasian, and HIV-positive. Being male and Caucasian is easy enough. At first, I hated being HIV positive because it exposed my other identity (that of a gay man). With time, however, I developed a stronger identity as an "HIV-positive person."

Worldwide, there are about 38 million HIV-positive people. Of all those people, a smaller number have progressed to AIDS. In the United States, well over 1 million people are HIV-positive. Again, a smaller number of those people have progressed to AIDS. If you're reading this book, you already know your HIV status. About one in four people in the U.S. don't know they have HIV. Now that you know, you can halt the progression to AIDS.

Here in the U.S., we call ourselves the *HIV community.* What's interesting about the HIV community is that members are wildly different, but we all share some of the same behaviors. If you're newly diagnosed with HIV, there's a 99 percent chance you got the virus—ultimately—from behavior related to drugs or sex. Whether you're a straight African-American female or you're a down-low Latino man, what we have in common is that—at some point—we had unsafe sex or used drugs.

Seeing the HIV community for what it is

How do we know that unsafe sex and injection drug use are the common denominator among people with HIV? The U.S. Centers for Disease Control and Prevention (also called the CDC) is the primary U.S. government agency that tracks statistics about HIV in the U.S. The CDC has monitored HIV trends by collecting information from thirty-three states since 2002. Not all states are included, so the estimates may not be perfect, but they are good enough that the CDC can see overall trends about risky behaviors, such as unsafe sex and substance abuse. According to the CDC:

GENDER OF PEOPLE WITH HIV

Male	74%
Female	26%

Females make up about one quarter of all people newly diagnosed with HIV.

AGE WHEN PEOPLE TEST HIV-POSITIVE

Younger than 13	less than 1%
13 to 24	13%
25 to 34	26%
35 to 44	34%
45 to 54	19%
55 to 64	5%
Older than 65	2%

This chart shows the age of people when they test positive for HIV. It does not show the age when people get the virus.

HOW MALES GET HIV

Male-to-male sexual contact	67%
Heterosexual (male-female) contact	15%
Injection drug use	13%
Male-to-male sexual contact and injection drug use	5%
Blood transfusions, hemophilia, perinatal, and risk not reported or identified	less than 1%

Over two-thirds of HIV-positive men can trace their infection to male-to-male sexual contact.

HOW FEMALES GET HIV

Heterosexual (male-female) contact	80%
Injection drug use	19%
Blood transfusions, hemophilia, perinatal, and risk not reported or identified	1%

As noted above, about one quarter of all new HIV infections are among women. Of these women, 80 percent can trace their infection to male-female sex.

RACES AND ETHNICITIES AMONG PEOPLE WITH HIV

African American	49%
Caucasian	31%
Latino	18%
Asian/Pacific Islander	1%
American Indian/Alaska Native	Less than 1%

About half of all new HIV infections are among African Americans. The majority are African-American males who had sexual contact with another male. The term *down low*—also known as DL—means "to keep something private," whether that refers to information or behavior. A man on the down low is having sexual contact with another man, but prefers to keep it a secret.

IN A SENTENCE:

If you're newly diagnosed with HIV, you can connect with others in the HIV community to help understand your identity as a person with HIV.

Talking about drugs, sex, and HIV

Tom Donahue was twenty-four years old when he tested positive for HIV. He was devastated at first, but gradually adjusted to the news. Living in rural Pennsylvania, Tom quickly discovered that people—friends, neighbors, community members—refused to discuss HIV and AIDS.

Tom's response was to launch a nonprofit organization called Who's Positive. A network of outspoken HIV-positive people, it provides information and support to young people, especially in high schools and colleges.

These days, Who's Positive organizes awareness campaigns for speakers at high schools and colleges (www.whospositive.com). One recent campaign consisted of a cross-country bus tour of HIV-positive young adults who gave speeches at various spots along the way.

Speaking around the country, one common question that Donahue gets asked is: Are you mad at the person who infected you? "Ultimately it was my responsibility to protect myself," says Donahue. "But then I found out that this person knew his status. He was just going through denial. He could have prevented it. That one moment of passion, of intimacy, of irresponsibility, changed my life forever. That's why I'm so passionate about reaching out to my peers about getting tested for HIV, so people know their status, it's empowering."

DAY 2

living

Adjusting to the News

CRYING IS a normal and healthy response after testing positive for HIV. Crying releases tension. In fact, studies show that crying brings down blood pressure, slows your heart rate, and relieves pressure on the cardiovascular system. The message: Let it all out.

"People who actually have access to their deep sadness and who are able to share it with others—these are probably rather healthy people," says Jelka Jonker, a therapist at AIDS Project Los Angeles.

Steve is a person who says he generally doesn't cry much. But he describes breaking down in tears after he tested HIV-positive. "I couldn't cry hard enough," he says.

On the other hand, some people feel emotionally numb at first. If you expected a positive test result, the news might bring a mixture of sadness and relief. The relief comes from finally knowing what you've suspected for some time. A positive test might feel like the last piece of a puzzle and now you can get on with dealing with reality.

Either way, there's a good chance you'll begin to feel nervous, overwhelmed, or even panicky. This feeling is called **anxiety**. People often deal with anxiety by using alcohol, food, prescription drugs, street drugs, and exercise.

Jonker says that it's important to feel the emotions, and not simply to block them with alcohol, drugs, or destructive behaviors. She says that you may need to "push through" these emotions as they happen. And there's no specific order as to how emotions will beset you. The emotional roller-coaster ride is quite normal—overwhelming at times, but quite normal.

Feeling nervous is normal

For better or worse, many people often rely on mind-altering substances to cope with stressful events in life. Few experiences are more stressful than discovering you have a potentially life-threatening disease such as HIV.

For some people, especially those who tend to be nervous or anxious in general, prescriptions drugs known as **sedatives** (Xanax, Ativan, or any benzodiazepine) might provide short-term relief from anxiety. However, if you're prone to substance abuse, sedatives or alcohol might hurt more than help your life in the long run.

There are a few healthier choices for initially coping with the news:

- ❍ **Cry.** Being weepy is for wimps. Try bawling with your heart and gut, like what you hear at an Italian funeral.
- ❍ **Comfort foods.** Forget the diet for now. Ice cream, macaroni and cheese, and pizza are generally considered comforting foods. But remember—comfort foods are just a short-term way to cope with difficult situations. A bad diet over time is not good for your health.
- ❍ **Walk, run, hike, or lift weights.** Studies show that regular exercisers adjust better and more quickly to the news of testing HIV-positive.
- ❍ **Creative endeavors.** Try writing or painting. Anything that takes your mind off things for a while—even a good movie—can be a great way to deal with scary feelings.

"The day I tested positive, my best friend brought over two canvasses and some oil paints," says Glenn G. "We sat for several hours and painted. I'm no painter, but I didn't care. Everything in my head was so frenetic and that's exactly what I painted. It got me through that day and that painting is still up on my wall today."

> *You'll probably experience some degree of anxiety, but that's completely normal and there are many ways to cope.*

learning

Beating Emotional Overload

TESTING POSITIVE for HIV can feel like a slow-motion car wreck for some people. In the hours afterward, you may have felt as though you were watching a movie and the diagnosis was given to someone in the movie. This experience is called **disassociation**. It's a fancy word for how your mind deals with traumatic events. Feeling "separate from yourself" is a normal reaction to very bad news.

For other people, the news is less traumatic. Daniel S. Berger, M.D., medical director at Northstar Healthcare, says that people today generally know that effective HIV medicine is available. He says some people might not even take the news seriously, thinking the diagnosis is on par with something like syphilis.

"Maybe they don't realize it in the beginning, but as time goes on, as they learn more about what it means to be infected, it hits them down the road," says Dr. Berger. "Sometimes they fall apart and sometimes they don't. At our clinic, we try to have newly diagnosed patients visit with a therapist to be evaluated to catch problems before they get out of hand."

Some people shut down entirely when they first get their HIV diagnosis. A study of people who were newly diagnosed with HIV showed that about one in three delay seeking medical attention for at least one year after their diagnosis. Another one-in-three people delay seeing a doctor for at least two years or more.

Denial is an option. It's possible to pretend nothing happened. If denial gets you through a particularly tough day, it can be a good thing. But over the course of weeks and months, using denial to cope with HIV will probably make things worse. Research also shows that people who use denial tend to progress faster to AIDS. I'm not saying that denial causes AIDS, but rather that denial can get in the way of your getting proper medical care.

Feel the feelings and talk about them

You will feel many different emotions in the first week after learning your HIV status. "It's usually helpful for people to talk to someone professionally to normalize all those feelings," says Jelka Jonker, a therapist at AIDS Project Los Angeles. She notes that people need to feel the emotions and experience the phases of adjustment.

Many people have gone through the same emotions and fears that you may be feeling right now. Some of the more common fears are:

○ **Fear of the unknown.** You might believe you won't live much longer.
○ **Fear of stigmatization.** You might think HIV will bring labeling, rejection, isolation, or discrimination.
○ **Concern about family.** You may be worried about the well-being of your children, parents, or close friends.
○ **Pressure to maintain a "false front."** You might feel as if you should act happy when you don't feel that way.

You might feel "on your own" with these worries or fears. You're not. Many people with HIV have experienced these thoughts. One way to manage your feelings is by talking with someone who has gone through similar experiences, or someone with professional training, such as an HIV counselor. Later in this book, I discuss in more detail how to find professional help, or at least how to connect with others in the same boat.

Self-blame is another common feeling

Self-blame is also a common feeling at first. You might have known how to avoid HIV but you didn't. This may lead to feelings of guilt or self-hate. "What goes through your mind is 'I should have used a condom' or 'I should have used a clean needle,'" says Mark H. "That whole woulda-shoulda-coulda thinking is completely understandable. The question to ask yourself now is: What am I going to do differently to stay healthy?"

"I'm the kind of person who always says, 'what if' or 'if only.' But I knew that it wouldn't help with HIV," say Rick G. "Try not to fall into this kind of thinking because it doesn't help you, it doesn't accomplish anything. The actions you take and your mental attitude all play a critical role in your health."

It's normal to feel remorse or guilt about some things from the past. After all, remorse and guilt help you make better decisions in the future—and that's a good thing. How many times do you touch a hot stove before you understand that it hurts?

Expect to feel bad at first about getting HIV. But if these feelings of guilt or self-blame eat away at you, or immobilize you for too long, they can get in the way of pursuing a healthier and happier future. Feel the feelings, understand that you can't change the past, and start making better choices in the days to come.

Anger is a normal response

"It's easier to feel anger than to feel shame, guilt, resentment, or sadness," says Mark H. "Sadness hurts, shame hurts, but anger doesn't hurt. You scream and yell and it somehow becomes someone else's problem."

You just found out you have HIV. One day, you're a regular person. The next day, you're different. What about other people who took part in unsafe behaviors? They didn't get the virus. Why did you get it?

Life isn't fair. Different things happen to different people. Sometimes these things make sense and sometimes they don't. If your best friend won a million dollars in the lottery, you might be a little jealous. In a similar way, you might feel angry with people who engaged in the same risky behaviors as you did but also tested negative for HIV. It's completely normal to feel this way.

For some people, this frustration may build up. Without really thinking about it, some people might blame their frustrations on people whom they actually care about. Some people might become angry with people who aren't going through the same thing, such as friends who have tested HIV-negative.

You may know the person who infected you—or least whom you suspect had a role in it. You may be angry with a spouse or a partner if you believe he or she infected you. It sounds strange, but you might even respond with anger to your spouse or partner if you believe *you* may have infected him or her.

It's normal to think about who infected you, or people whom you may have infected. However, confronting that person is not a great idea during the first week. Unless you're prepared to deal with the consequences of such an exchange now, consider taking some time to adjust to the news for yourself.

In the end, you'll probably find that most of your anger is directed at yourself. If you're the type of person who tends toward self-destructive behavior, you might be compelled to continue engaging in those behaviors. This is to be expected. But eventually you'll get tired of hurting yourself. At some point, the pain of hurting yourself will be greater than the pain of forgiving yourself. When you're ready, there's plenty of help out there.

IN A SENTENCE:

Shock, self-blame, and anger are all common feelings at first.

Protecting Your Privacy

GREG M. PREFERS to keep his last name private. Living in a small town in North Carolina, he doesn't advertise his HIV status. He learned of his diagnosis after applying for a $100,000 life-insurance policy.

"The insurance company sent me a letter saying they declined my coverage due to some abnormal blood work, but they didn't say what it was," says Greg M. "They said if I would sign some papers, the results would be sent to my physician."

That's exactly what happened. After Greg's doctor got the results from the insurance company, she scheduled a new test, saying she didn't trust insurance companies. Ultimately, Greg's own doctor confirmed the diagnosis.

Doctors and patients alike harbor mistrust of the insurance industry—and with good reason. Insurance companies can be unscrupulous as they routinely deny life and health insurance to people with HIV. Another common mistrust is that of the government, which has its own dubious record when dealing with health and minorities.

People with HIV should be concerned about two types of privacy: medical and community. *Medical privacy* is having the right to know about which private companies or government agencies have your name on file as HIV-positive. *Community privacy* refers to the people physically around you. You have the right to know whom in your family and community knows that you have HIV.

Medical privacy is a right, but there's a price to pay for it

In 2006, the U.S. Centers for Disease Control and Prevention (CDC) announced sweeping new rules about how people should be tested in the U.S. The CDC is a federal agency that aims to prevent and control infectious and chronic diseases. The CDC rules encourage hospitals and doctors around the country to routinely offer an HIV tests to all patients between the ages of thirteen and sixty-four. The rules also give guidelines that relate to your medical records.

The CDC new rules hinge on what's called *name-based reporting*. This type of reporting means that when you test positive, your name gets reported to the government. In a perfect world, your name would privately go from your doctor to your local health department, then to the CDC. As it stands now, the CDC creates one master list of names and related statistics from only thirty-three of fifty states. The CDC wants to get a better estimate of how many Americans have HIV. Also, these statistics justify federal programs for HIV medicine and health care in the form of Medicaid, Medicare, and funding for the Ryan White Comprehensive AIDS Resources Emergency Act.

The Ryan White AIDS Emergency Act is a law that Congress passed in 1990. It provides money to individual states to help pay for health care for people with HIV and AIDS. But in 2004, there were over 45 million uninsured people in the U.S. HIV-positive people are routinely denied health insurance. Ultimately, Ryan White funding covers the cost of health care for people who can't get insurance in the first place. Ultimately, the CDC and a few individual states are fighting over who's footing the bill for health care.

The CDC is asking individual states to adopt the rules as law. All fifty individual states have their own laws related to HIV and AIDS. Often these state laws contradict the federal rules. For example, the state governments of the District of Columbia and Maryland are now debating whether to obey the new CDC rules. California and Illinois are two other states that do not yet conform to the CDC rules. Local counties or health departments often have added layers of other laws or policies.

Opponents of name-based reporting say that the federal government might use the information in a malicious way, in ways that could infringe on constitutional rights to privacy. Still, if the states don't follow the federal rules, they may lose substantial Ryan White money. Time will tell.

Meanwhile, if you live in the U.S., you should expect your HIV test results to be documented in your *medical record,* along with your *informed consent* form (which means that you agreed to take an HIV test). If you find yourself in an emergency room, a hospital, or an STD clinic, you can expect that anyone who has access to your medical record also has access to your HIV status. But remember that the laws and policies vary from state to state. You can find more information by calling the AIDS Hotline in your particular state. More information is listed in the Resources Guide at the end of this book.

Even if the federal government does nothing suspicious with its master list of HIV names, accidents and breaches in security just happen. In 2006, a worker in a Florida health department inadvertently e-mailed out the names of more than 6,600 local people with AIDS and HIV. The incident resulted from simple human error.

Privacy in your community is important

For many people with HIV, it's hard to keep a life-changing secret—me included. I work for a software company in Los Angeles, California. I have three coworkers who know my HIV status: two because I purposely told them, and the other ran across this book in a bookstore. Most people at work probably don't care much either way.

On the other hand, I tend hide my HIV status from my neighbors that live in my building. The only exception is one neighbor; she just earned a medical degree specializing in HIV among children. Just recently, in the hallway, we were quietly talking about something related to HIV. Suddenly, a door swung open and another neighbor appeared. When he walked by us, we all chatted as good neighbors should. He said he wasn't feeling well— and then innocently said, "at least I don't have AIDS."

Living in Los Angeles, I was surprised to hear that comment. If I were in a different situation, I might see the intended humor. Still, I overlooked the incident in exchange for maintaining friendly neighbors.

Across the country not far from Durham, North Carolina, Greg's experience with HIV privacy is very different. He works for a pest control company where he visits up to thirty homes a day to perform his job. He wonders what his customers might think. "If they found out I had HIV, I don't know whether they would let me back in their house or not." When I interviewed him over the phone, we chuckled at irony of working in "pest" control.

As for other areas of his life, Greg M. feels frustration about being so guarded in his own community. "I can't pray out loud because I'm scared somebody's going to hear me praying about the HIV and get scared of me, run out of the church," he says. "I'm in a Pentecostal church, so I don't want to be cast out or ostracized. The religion I believe in, they believe in Sodom and Gomorrah, and that's the way I was brought up. That's all I know.

"I've been preached to that God doesn't like homosexuals, and stuff like that. If I had told anybody in my family when I was coming up and going to school that I was gay, they would have hung me out, they'd have thrown rocks at me. So you have to hide behind the bushes."

Even with his secrets, he still attends church faithfully. "I read a lot, tried to find out as much as I could. I prayed a lot and started going back to church." Although he keeps his prayers private, he says, "I think God loves everybody."

Putting aside the true intentions of a supreme being, be aware that your community—the people in your family, your neighbors, friends, fellow workers or students, religious and spiritual groups—they all have a profound effect on your life. Sometimes that effect is good, sometimes not. Either way, you always have the right to HIV privacy in your own community.

If you ask me, however, giving up some privacy in the form of the CDC's name-based reporting makes sense. With a few good watchdogs and activists on the lookout for abuse or negligence by state and federal officials, the plan could have huge benefits for the entire country.

IN A SENTENCE:

> *You have the right to "HIV privacy," but the specifics of those rights depend on your state or community.*

learning

Healthy Choices Make Healthy People

I'M IN the car with my HIV-positive friend Allen G., and he's driving way too fast. As he speeds and weaves recklessly between lanes, I'm trying to talk to him about HIV. He turns to me—of course ignoring the road in front of us—and says, "I drive too fast to worry about HIV."

As his passenger, I have to agree. I do think it's more likely he'll die from a car accident than from AIDS. In fact, a new study of people with HIV shows that the likelihood of dying from AIDS has decreased by 55 percent. This is good news for all of us. But the study also revealed that the likelihood of HIV-positive people dying from *something else* also has increased by nearly one-third.

The success of new HIV treatments is clear in this study. But the researchers also noted that people with HIV, at least in developed countries, are not immune to "common conditions" that affect the rest of the population. The top causes include heart disease, garden-variety cancer, and substance abuse—all of which are treatable when caught early or preventable with appropriate lifestyle changes.

For Allen G., my friend who's reckless behind the wheel, a smart lifestyle change would be to improve his driving. But for the rest of us with HIV, a wise move is learning what potential health risks may be a challenge in the future. Armed with this knowledge, we can make better lifestyle choices to prevent or minimize those risks.

If you are newly diagnosed with HIV, the future may seem a bit scary. The road in front of you may seem unfamiliar. You'll need to make count-less choices as you move forward. But take comfort in knowing that being healthy with HIV is similar to being healthy as a human being. And when you encounter a difficult choice about your health, also know that are a few techniques to help you make better decisions.

Live like a healthy person and you'll probably become one

How do you live like a healthy person? One day at a time. For example, each day you choose the kind of food that you eat for breakfast. You can choose a slice of cake with potato chips. Or, you can choose whole-grain cereal with fruit. Now, imagine that you made the same choice everyday for ten years. Over time, your choices would add up and affect your heart, which affects your health, which affects your life. Use your brain to make better choices and you'll probably get better health.

"Lead the same sort of general healthy life that you would if you wanted to be in the top 10 percent of healthy people." This is the advice to people with HIV offered by Anthony Fauci, M.D., director of the National Insti-tute of Allergy and Infectious Diseases (NIAID). Fauci is one of the top "thinkers" in the in the areas of HIV, both as a scientist and as the direc-tor of NIAID.

According to Fauci, the top-five things that healthy people do are:

○ stop smoking
○ exercise regularly
○ eat nutritiously
○ avoid recreational drugs
○ get enough sleep

If you have HIV, Fauci gives a few more suggestions:

○ get a physician or health provider with whom you're comfortable
○ never hesitate to get a second opinion
○ be compulsive about follow-up care
○ lead a generally healthy life

If you're newly diagnosed with HIV, the overall message is clear: Take excellent care of yourself. Of course, having HIV is a major health challenge. But new HIV treatments are making this condition far less worrisome. Instead, redirect some of your energy to consider your life as a whole. Like my HIV-positive friend who drives recklessly, HIV is probably not the biggest threat to his current well being. As I suggested to my friend Allen G.: slow down and think about the choices you make.

"Reframing" your situation can help you make better choices

One way that mental health professionals help their patients make better choices is by using a technique called *reframing*. Therapists and psychologists use reframing to coach their patients into thinking about certain situations in a whole new way.

An easy way to understand the concept of reframing is to think about a frame around a picture. Depending on what is "framed" in a picture, you will have a certain amount of information about what's happening. A painter who is painting a particular landscape, for example, might only frame a tree or a house. By framing, the painter determines what you will see of the entire landscape.

In your mind, frames influence the way you understand and think about a situation. Frames establish the borders of what you think about. What's in your frame is important and present in your thoughts. What's out of your frame is unimportant and out of your thoughts.

If you've recently been diagnosed with HIV, it may feel like you're being attacked by the virus. Your mental frame might be filled with thoughts of HIV and its consequences. If you were to visually draw your feelings on a piece of paper, it might look something like the following:

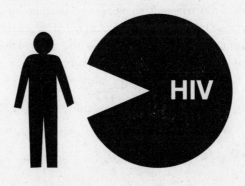

In your mental frame, you can imagine yourself as the human figure here. The challenges of HIV might look something like a giant PacMan that's about to swallow you. But don't forget about the other things in your life, things that might deserve more attention.

When Allen G. declared that he drives too fast to worry about HIV, he was reframing his perception of his health risks. For example, Allen's mental frame would look something like the following:

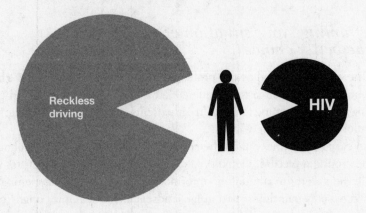

New research clearly suggests that people with HIV also need to reframe their own risk perceptions as well. According to this research, people with HIV are living longer in a good state of health. As such, new problems are emerging. These problems include overeating and smoking cigarettes—both of which can lead to bigger problems down the road and both of which are preventable with lifestyle changes.

Reframing your situation can help you step back to see the bigger picture. With this bigger view of your health situation, you can make better choices over time.

Now that you know about some of the basics of making better choices, does it mean that you will quit smoking and become an exercise fanatic tomorrow? Of course not. Radical changes in behavior are difficult and rarely are sustained over time. But what you can do now is begin to understand that HIV is only one piece of a larger puzzle. That puzzle is you being at your healthiest, you being at your best. It all starts with one good choice today.

This is your brain making better choices

A healthy brain makes better choices. "When your brain doesn't work right, you don't work right," writes Daniel G. Amen, M.D., a psychiatrist, brain imaging specialist, and medical director of Amen Clinics, which specializes in brain health. In his book, *How to Make a Good Brain Great,* he outlines a number of ways to improve your own brain health:

○ Think about your brain everyday. Think about how it feels and operates. And when you think about your brain, make an effort to think good thoughts.
○ Protect your brain from injury, toxins such as drugs and alcohol, and too much stress. Treat your brain like a good friend.
○ Get enough sleep.
○ Eat nutritiously, but don't overeat.
○ Consider supplements such as omega-3 fatty acids and fish oils.
○ Get enough exercise. What's good for your heart is also good for your brain.
○ Learn new things and have experiences that you wouldn't ordinarily seek out. For example, try to practice writing with your other hand.
○ Listen to classical music, which seems to help the brain's wiring.
○ Get mental help when needed.

IN A SENTENCE:

The first step to being healthy with HIV is simply being a healthy person in general.

DAY 4

living

Overcoming Stigma and Shame

FOR MANY people, HIV is a mark of disgrace. However, the disgrace is in the judgment, not in the disease. The word *stigma* means a "mark of discredit." It comes from an older word, *stigmata*, which is used to describe the wounds of a crucifix. *HIV stigma* refers to the prejudice against, discounting of, discrediting of, and discrimination against people who are perceived to have and do have HIV, as well as anyone associated with them.

In everyday life, HIV stigma could mean being excluded from employer health insurance, rejection by friends, workplace gossip, or even violence. What's fueling the stigma may be the persistence of inaccurate information. For example, a recent study found that many Americans still express false beliefs and discomfort about people with HIV and AIDS. The study polled a sample of Americans, and it found that:

○ 41 percent believed they could get AIDS from using public toilets
○ 50 percent believed that they could get AIDS from being coughed on
○ 50 percent believed they could get AIDS by sharing a drinking glass
○ 33 percent believed that AIDS can be contracted by donating blood

HIV is not transmitted through any of these ways.

On the bright side, the study also noted that the percentage of Americans who actively avoid people with AIDS is shrinking. Support for extremely coercive policies such as mass quarantine of people with the virus has declined dramatically: Only 12 percent in 1999 agreed that people with AIDS should be separated from the rest of society, compared to 34 percent in 1991.

"The belief that AIDS is easily spread and that people with AIDS should be blamed for their illness are important ingredients of stigma," says Gregory M. Herek, a professor of psychology at the University of California at Davis, who conducted the poll of Americans.

"In the early years of the epidemic, most AIDS information programs stressed that AIDS can't be spread through casual contact such as sharing a drinking glass or being around someone who is sneezing," he said. "It's clear that we need to revive those messages and keep reminding people how AIDS is and isn't transmitted."

"Anytime you're around something for the first time, you're frightened," says Rosetta M. She compares the HIV stigma to that of genital herpes. "One in five Americans has genital herpes, but no one knows anyone with herpes. Now, 'one in five' is more popular than Nike—and we all know someone who owns a pair of Nikes."

As with herpes, society views HIV as a "sex" issue, not necessarily a "health" issue. "If I went out and got in a car accident and I got a scar, people can look past it. But if I go out and have sex and something happens, people look differently at that." Rosetta M. contends that many people with HIV have internalized these negative messages, which ultimately leads to feelings of shame.

Shame is bad for your health

Imagine walking into a room full of people who were afraid to touch you. That's how it feels sometimes for people with HIV. You may have a strong defense against the stigma at first, but with time, the negative messages might sink in, and fuel personal feelings of shame.

Shame is a painful emotion caused by guilt, shortcomings, or behaving improperly. According to Jelka Jonker, stigma and shame are especially prevalent among women and the Latino community. "This can happen because [HIV-positive people] are married, bisexual, or gay." Being gay is more difficult within Latino culture, she said. "So there's a lot of stigma there, and HIV is hard to talk about it."

You might feel shame or embarrassment when talking about HIV. This is understandable. But when that shame keeps you from seeking medical care, not letting go of shame will work against you. The challenge, says Rosetta M., is knowing when to cut loose the shame, which she says was probably there even before the HIV diagnosis. She says that for some people, HIV has been a catalyst for confronting feelings of shame. When she tested positive, her motto was: Sink or swim. "I think most of our natures are to swim, even if we only doggie paddle."

IN A SENTENCE:

> *Be prepared to experience stigma or feel shame about your HIV status, which can stem from old, deep-seated feelings that predate your diagnosis or public ignorance about your condition.*

learning

Religion, God, Faith and Spirituality

THINK OF spirituality and religion as two different circles on a piece of paper. For some people, the circles intersect and overlap. For other people, the two circles couldn't be farther apart. However, what we all have in common is a body, a mind, and a soul.

Obviously, the body is the physical stuff—skin, muscles, bones, and even the genes that were passed along from our parents. The mind is the ability to think, to add numbers, to remember a birthday, and to run from danger, for example, when being chased by a snarling dog.

But the soul, well, that's everything else. It's outside the realm of science and intellect. The soul is the spark of life, the life force, the spirit that makes us want to love, hope for better things, honor truth, or offer compassion. In fact, observing, appreciating, and caring for one's spirit is why many people use the term *spirituality*.

When you initially test positive for HIV, it may feel as if your spirit has been hurt. It's true that your body may be under attack by the virus. Your mind may be in overdrive cranking out scary thoughts. But your spirit is more resistant because it's larger, in a sense, than both your mind and your body.

When you protect your spirit, when you nurture it, or when you show compassion toward yourself, you are being spiritual. It doesn't mean you are being religious or that you believe in God—especially one with a white beard who guards the pearly gates of heaven. For many people, being spiritual can mean being good to yourself in a way that seems to defy reason or the laws of physics.

"I do meditation," says Tim L., who is HIV-positive. He considers himself spiritual but doesn't have an opinion, one way or the other, about God. "I do 'positive reinforcement' of my mental attitude, which is more like a mantra. It depends on the situation."

He positions himself in a relaxed position, maybe against a couch or in a hot bath. "I'll say to myself certain things like 'my mind, body, heart, and soul are in perfect balance,' or 'every day in every way I get better and better,'" he says.

"There's a positive energy in you that needs to be released," says Tim L. "I accept and use my own healing power. I've seen the healing power that people have inside themselves, so I know it's there. I give myself the permission to tap into it, to release it, and to accept it."

Accepting the idea of a healing power within one's self might at first seem foreign or unnatural. But for many people, relying upon such a power within can be a force in coping with HIV.

Faith in God is a healing power for many people

"I believe in God," say Donald W., who is an HIV counselor for the Eastern Regional AIDS Resource Consultation Center in Norfolk, Virginia. He was diagnosed with HIV in 1990, and then diagnosed with chronic hepatitis C several years later. Today, he's a recovering addict, a husband, and a father of two sons. He's also here to send a message to others: If you want to survive, use any means necessary. For Donald W., one of those means is a faith in God.

"Faith has a major role in my life," says Donald W. But it wasn't always that way. Growing up, religion played a superficial role at best. "When I went to church, it was like for Easter—to be dressed up and to been seen."

It was not until many years, after a severe drug addiction and bouts with depression, that Donald W. would begin to build a solid spiritual foundation. "When I went into the rooms of Narcotics Anonymous—which is a spiritual program—we read the twelve steps and the twelve traditions. I kept hearing about a 'power greater than ourselves, a God as we understood him.'" This, for Donald W., would soon become a stepping-stone to the Catholic Church.

So what role does spirituality have in helping people cope with HIV? Perhaps a more objective question is: What are the risks and the benefits of pursuing a path of spirituality?

Faith is a two-way street

In a recent article in the *Journal of the American Medical Association*, Harold G. Koenig, M.D., associate professor of psychiatry and associate professor of medicine at Duke University Medical Center, attempted to shed light on some of these questions.

Pointing to a review of published studies, 66 percent found a "statistically significant relationship between religious involvement and better mental health, greater social support, or less substance abuse."

According to Koenig, many patients have little control over their health conditions, which creates anxiety and, in some cases, furious attempts to regain control. When such attempts fail, anxiety worsens and depression develops. Religious beliefs and practices can provide an indirect form of control that helps to interrupt this vicious cycle. "They enable a patient to turn a health situation over to God and stop worrying and obsessing about it," writes Koenig.

For Precious J., a treatment advocate for Women Alive, an AIDS service organization in Los Angeles, faith has played a critical role in helping her cope with her diagnosis. "It helped me get past the anger," she says, referring specifically to an ex-boyfriend who, she says, infected her with the virus. "With the support of my mom, prayer, going to church, that really helped. I believe—I know—that's why I'm here today, because of my faith in God."

As part of her spiritual evolution, she also points out that faith alone is not enough. "You have to take responsibility for your actions. I just couldn't put all the blame on my ex-boyfriend. I willingly laid down with him without making him put on a condom. That's the part I played in it. I didn't protect myself. I had to get over that part."

Blaming God won't help resolve the problem

Rick G. was twenty-eight years old when he learned his HIV status and doubted he'd reach the age of thirty. "But I had such faith, such good friends, and the love of my family—even though my family didn't know I was HIV-positive. They all kept me going."

According to Rick G., not everyone who had faith before diagnosis maintains it; some people may not be capable of accepting responsibility themselves. "If you can blame God, it takes it out of your hands. This way, you not only get to be the victim, but the angry victim. Sometimes when people feel helpless, they turn to anger to make themselves feel less helpless. The problem is that while you're flailing about in anger, you're still helpless. And those angry people just don't see that."

In the end, everyone eventually wakes up to the same question: How is blame going to help me? How is getting angry with God going to help me out of this? How is blaming myself going to help? Only when you move past blame, Rick G. says, do you begin the process of emotional healing.

Faith is not a substitute for medical care

What's not helpful is when religious beliefs conflict with appropriate medical care. Studies of people with HIV have shown that some stop taking their medications or fail to seek medical care on religious grounds. Religious activities like prayer have been used instead of traditional medical care to treat illness. This situation poses larger dilemmas for physicians who monitor patients.

According to Koenig, even if religious beliefs conflict with medical care—as those of Jehovah's Witnesses or Christian Scientists—physicians should be cautious about rejecting them. Instead, he suggests that physicians try to understand the patient's worldview by beginning a dialogue that shows respect for the beliefs and a willingness to work with the patient.

Donald W. concurs, citing a number of philosophical differences that come between his church and his health. "I was fortunate enough to find a church that had an HIV support group. I disagreed with some things that were said there early on and still do. They would say things like, 'Have faith and stop taking your medicine.' I would say, 'Have you lost your mind?'"

As part of Donald W.'s job, he's often asked to speak about AIDS at schools and churches, which often balk at certain topics. "They say, 'no condoms, don't talk about sex.' They want me only to quote the scripture. Let's get real, people are having sex—all through the Bible belt."

Recent surveys have shown that the southeastern region of the United States is the new epicenter of the HIV epidemic. Why? According to Donald W., the reason is primarily the denial about the prevalence of sexual activity and substance abuse "especially in the churches." He said the overriding mantra in the Bible belt is silence, except for abstinence. "That's the philosophy down here: You shouldn't be doing it."

Religion-based denial is compounding the problems

Bob Munk is a seasoned HIV advocate and the driving force behind New Mexico's AIDS InfoNet, an online information Web site. He's concerned that climbing rates of HIV infection in the southeast United States are an ominous sign for the region.

The trend, he says, is just part of the stigma that surrounds HIV, especially in the Southeast, where the infrastructure of AIDS service organizations pales in comparison to the region's religion-based infrastructure.

He says religion-based denial "plays into people not wanting to get tested. If they do get tested, they don't want to get treated or to disclose. They don't disclose, so they don't realize that everybody around them has probably got the virus."

It's exactly this sense of isolation that drives Donald W. to continue being outspoken about HIV and substance-abuse issues despite the obstacles. It's his faith, he says, that keeps him moving forward. "I wake up every morning. I do my meds. I believe in God. I truly believe in God," says Donald W. "He's walked me through this so far, and he's not finished with me yet."

IN A SENTENCE:

> *Relying upon spiritual tools—whether they are religious in nature or not—can be an effective way of coping with HIV.*

DAY 5

living

Free Services
Are Available

YOU MIGHT need some help. You might want some advice about health insurance. Maybe you're having problems with your landlord or you need a lawyer. Perhaps you have a toothache but you can't afford to see a dentist right now. In these cases, the HIV system—sometimes called AIDS organizations—can be a big help.

Equally, the HIV system can seem intimidating at first. These organizations are often highly bureaucratic. Call an AIDS organization and you'll probably get put on hold, transferred a few times, and end up having to leave a voice message.

"The system is enormously frustrating, but cracking the system has saved my life," says Mark H. "Many states have special programs that offer free HIV medicine or affordable health insurance."

AIDS organizations offer special—and often free—services to people with HIV, but to become affiliated with one in your area often requires some persistence on your part and plenty of paperwork. If you need professional services sooner rather than later, start the paperwork as soon as possible.

How do you start? Call your state's HIV hotline. A list of state hotlines can be found in the Resources Guide at the end of this book. Start on a local level. Look to see what organizations are in your neighborhood or in your city. Then talk with people in those organizations to find out more.

"It all falls back on your own research," says Mark H. "There's not a state in our country where you can't find some resource to help. The Internet is a great source of information. If you don't have access to the Internet, you can always pick up the phone, even if you're in Wyoming."

At least in the larger metropolitan areas, here are some free or low-cost services:

- ○ **Referrals for you and significant others**. Say a family member discovers you have HIV and becomes extremely distressed. You may need to find an appropriate counselor for this family member.
- ○ **Assistance with healthcare or prescription drugs**. Many states offer free or discounted programs to help people without health insurance. A case manager may be able to find various options for you.
- ○ **Dental care**. Often overlooked, dental care is critical for maintaining the overall health of people with HIV. Unfortunately, dental insurance is not easy to find. Many AIDS organizations provide dental services or offer access to special programs.
- ○ **Nutrition education and dieticians.** Free or discounted consultations with trained nutrition experts or registered dieticians are provided by many AIDS organizations. Nutrition is especially important if you're thinking about starting on HIV medicine.
- ○ **Legal assistance.** Say your health insurance company suddenly decides not to pay a $5,000 medical bill. A lawyer may be able to help you force the company to pay the claim or at least negotiate an acceptable repayment plan.
- ○ **Events and workshops.** Many AIDS organizations offer local seminars or presentations on new medicine, emerging side effects, safe sex, dating, or social events.
- ○ **Mental health services.** Perhaps you received the news of your HIV diagnosis amid other stressful life events. The compounding issues may cause you to be depressed or extremely nervous. Discussing these feelings with a trained therapist can help you work through some of the emotional issues.
- ○ **Support groups.** Support groups are usually safe places to discuss in detail how to cope with day-to-day worries that come with having HIV.
- ○ **Substance-abuse counseling.** Perhaps you've been experimenting with illicit drugs such as crystal meth and you're having trouble

quitting. For some people, HIV may be secondary to substance abuse. Drug counseling is available to help with these issues.

○ **Safe, stable, and affordable housing.** If you have children, finding appropriate housing may be a concern for you. Some AIDS organizations offer help in finding low-income housing.

○ **Political representation**. It may not seem important to you now, but it's good to know that people are looking out for the rights of people with HIV as a whole. Money for HIV services and research often comes from Congress, so it's good to know that you are being represented on a political level.

More details about the services offered by AIDS organizations are discussed later in this book. If you suddenly find yourself in an emergency, consider jumping ahead for more information.

IN A SENTENCE:

> *Cracking the AIDS organization system can be difficult and frustrating, but it has enormous benefits.*

learning

Frequently Asked Questions

What is HIV?

HIV is a nothing more than a virus. The term *HIV* is the abbreviation for *Human Immunodeficiency Virus*. In the 1980s, scientists gave it the "Human" part of its name because only humans can contract HIV. Animals can't get it and you can't get it from animals. However, some viruses are similar to HIV. These unique viruses can infect monkeys and cats. But don't worry; these particular viruses can't be transmitted to people. And you can't infect your pet cat with HIV.

Scientists believe that a long time ago HIV was a very different virus, one that infected only chimpanzees. Because humans ate chimpanzees for food in rural areas of Africa, eventually the virus learned how to survive in humans. In fact, scientists believe the jump from chimp to human happened between 1926 and 1946. The virus probably didn't spread much because people in these rural communities had limited contact with larger cities.

In the 1960s, people from rural African communities began to migrate to large cities. During this time, the incidence of sexually transmitted diseases, including HIV, accelerated and spread throughout Africa. In fact, old blood samples from a man who lived in the Congo showed that he had died from AIDS-related complications in 1959. HIV found its way to the United States around 1978 as world travel became more common.

What's the difference between HIV and AIDS?

HIV is a virus that infects the immune system and slowly damages it over time. Someone who has tested positive for infection with HIV is referred to as *HIV-positive*. AIDS is a collection of severe illnesses, which occurs when someone has a damaged immune system. Without medicine, many HIV-positive people do go on to develop AIDS, but this usually takes eight to eleven years, depending on the individual.

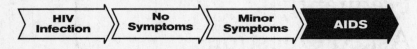

Is HIV the cause of AIDS?

In case you have any doubts, HIV is the cause of AIDS. *AIDS* stands for *Acquired Immune Deficiency Syndrome*. It's "acquired" because you have to get it somehow. It's not genetic and can't be passed down from generation to generation. The way people transmit HIV is through blood, semen, pre-cum, vaginal fluids, menstrual blood, and breast milk. You cannot get HIV through, saliva, sweat, urine, or feces.

The "Immune Deficiency" part of the name describes how HIV attacks the human immune system. The virus weakens the immune system to the point where other infections and cancers—that ordinarily wouldn't have a chance to make you sick—now have the opportunity to do damage. Doctors call these infections and cancers *opportunistic infections.*

The "Syndrome" part of AIDS describes the fact that AIDS isn't really a disease in a strict medical sense—it is a syndrome, a collection of symptoms. These symptoms are caused by an underlying condition: a weak immune system due to HIV infection. In theory, no one has ever died of AIDS itself. Rather, people die from opportunistic infections that flourish when the immune system is crippled.

Some people doubt that HIV causes AIDS. Me? I have no doubt whatsoever that HIV is what causes AIDS. Even if you put the science aside, I've seen the proof in my own life. Over the years, I've been on and off medicine. When my HIV is fully suppressed by medicine, I feel better and healthier. When the virus is not suppressed by medicine, I feel tired and I get sick. For me, the proof is in my daily life.

What are the symptoms of HIV?

Without medical intervention, HIV progresses along a predictable course. Within one to three weeks after infection with virus, most people experience flulike symptoms, such as fever, sore throat, headache, skin rash, swollen lymph nodes, and a vague feeling of discomfort. These symptoms can last one to four weeks. This initial phase is known as *acute infection*. During this time, HIV reproduces rapidly in the blood and circulates throughout the body. The immune system kicks in and reduces the virus at first, but it can't eliminate it. After acute infection, people usually experience a several-year period without any symptoms at all.

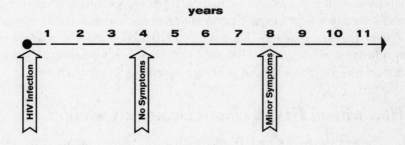

Is HIV a punishment for bad behavior?

Many people believe that HIV is a "punishment" for bad behavior. Studies of people show that "attributing one's HIV status as a 'punishment'" is a common clinical response. Ultimately, the HIV is just a tiny piece of genetic material. There are 1,000 to 1,500 different types of viruses in the world. Of these, about 250 types cause some disease in humans, including the common cold virus. Now, do you believe that getting a cold is a punishment? Animals get viruses that are similar to HIV. Do you believe that the animals are being punished? Every day, babies are born with HIV. Do you believe that newborns are being punished?

Viruses are found in virtually all forms of life—humans, animals, plants, and even bacteria. HIV just happens to survive best in humans. Once implanted in the human population, the virus just hopped from one person to the next. That's the reality.

Now, how you want to interpret that reality is entirely up to you. Maybe you haven't thought about it. Maybe you're not sure. Maybe it just seems like getting HIV is a punishment. And of course, some people in society will insist that HIV is a punishment. But it's not. It's just a virus. If you believe those people, at least remember that it's your choice to believe what they say and it's your choice to continue punishing yourself.

Am I stupid for getting HIV?

It's understandable that some people might feel "stupid" for getting HIV. Society has a way of making people feel bad for some behaviors. But remember, it's not an issue of intelligence, but rather it's a matter of benefits and consequences. HIV is a consequence for a behavior. Along with any behavior also comes a consequence. If you engaged in risky behaviors, you'll need to take responsibility for your actions. You may need to let go of idea that "someone else" has given you HIV. You engaged in a behavior that resulted in you getting HIV. So, you aren't stupid for getting HIV, you just took a risk. The hard part is being responsible for your actions.

How will an HIV diagnosis change my sex life?

After testing positive for HIV, the vast majority of men and women eventually continue to be sexually active. However, in the first week or month, it's normal to avoid sex. Some even consider celibacy, saying they will "never have sex again." In the first few months after testing HIV-positive, sex may seem awkward for you or your partner. You might feel "dirty" or unattractive to other people, and these feelings may come and go. Eventually, most people learn to enjoy safe sex and adjust. But it's also important to understand that you now have a responsibility to not put other people at risk. It is your responsibility to ensure that your sex or drug partners do not get HIV. It is possible to infect someone by having unsafe sex or sharing needles and you need to know that.

Does alternative therapy help with HIV?

No, alternative therapies do not specifically fight HIV. Many studies have attempted to prove that alternative medicine improves HIV. By all accounts, they have failed to show a positive connection. Some alternative therapies are dangerous and can make HIV worse. However, if you're looking for ways to reduce stress, anxiety, or depression, chances are much better you'll find some alternative therapies beneficial. Some forms of alternative therapy that may improve stress and anxiety include yoga, massage, meditation, and acupuncture.

Why should I trust doctors or pharmaceutical companies?

This requires a two-part answer: First, by trusting your doctor, you get the benefit of receiving health care, which can help you live longer and healthier. The second part of the answer is: You probably should not trust most pharmaceutical companies. It's doesn't mean these companies are bad, it only means that they are motivated by profit, not by social causes. It's always helpful to understand this agenda when reading brochures and pamphlets produced by pharmaceutical companies.

IN A SENTENCE:

> *Many people have the same questions when they first discover they have HIV.*

DAY 6

living

Meeting Others
in the Same Boat

"I'VE NEVER really been much of the support-group type," says Rick G. "Instead, a bunch of us HIV-positive guys get together on Thursday evenings at a bar in Chicago called Berlin. We usually meet after work, have a couple of drinks, and talk.

"In fact, one evening we talked about support groups," says Rick G. "We decided meeting here was the closest thing we have to a support group. Basically, we all have plenty of friends, we have family, and people that we can talk with."

In the first few days, weeks, and months after testing HIV-positive, talking about HIV might not be easy for you. You might not be ready to discuss the issue with your family or certain friends. On the other hand, you might feel isolated and alone.

If you don't know anyone with HIV, one option is attending a short-term support group. Many local health or AIDS organizations offer support groups. Many of these groups are tailored to different needs—such as spiritual guidance and recovery issues—and different populations—such as gay men, women, people of African descent, people of Latino descent, young adults, and family members. Some groups even offer an "HIV buddy" program where newly diagnosed individuals can talk with HIV-positive people of similar backgrounds.

On a more scientific level, here's what some studies say about support groups:

○ Support groups were superior to standard psychotherapy among HIV-positive men with depressed moods.
○ 86 percent of support group participants (men and women) showed significant improvements in "distress severity."
○ Support groups may help people living with HIV maintain safe sexual practices and guide individuals in making positive behavioral changes.

"Don't just go to any support group," warns Rick G. "Shop around. Find out about the organizations that offer these groups. If a support group is sponsored by a hospital, maybe that's too cold and clinical for you. If the group is organized by a nonprofit organization, you might think it's too touchy-feely for you. If you don't like the people in the group, don't go. Find another way."

How to connect with a local AIDS service organization

Finding an AIDS service organization (ASO) in your area is easy. The hard part is dealing with all the paperwork involved. Here's a step-by-step list of how to connect with an ASO:

○ At the end of this book, you'll find a Resource Guide of ASOs. These organizations provide services that are paid for by the Ryan White AIDS Emergency Act. Most ASOs offer some type of support group for people who are newly diagnosed with HIV.
○ Find an ASO near you. If there are many to choose from, try picking one that most closely matches what you are looking for.
○ First call the ASO or look online for more information. You might call an organization only to get an answering machine or a message. You might be asked to leave a name and number for a return call back. It may be difficult to leave your name on a machine at first, but remember there are benefits for you.
○ If you don't get a call back from an ASO within about a week, you'll need to call again. Some ASO are small and sometimes disorganized or understaffed. Call back, leave several messages, and always be persistent.

HIV

IN A SENTENCE:

> *Talking with other people in similar situations can help you come to terms with your own situation.*

learning

Cleaning Needles

LET'S FACE it, some people use needles to administer legal and illegal drugs or hormones. If those people have HIV, it's possible that HIV and other viruses can linger in blood droplets inside the used needles. If these needles are shared, it's possible to infect another person. Many states ban the sale of needles without a prescription. Unable to legally access clean needles, some people reuse them or get used ones from unreliable sources.

Needle-exchange programs are simply programs where clean needles are exchanged for dirty ones. The purpose of this is to prevent the sharing of needles or injection equipment, which prevents HIV and other diseases. Many programs also offer services to participants of needle exchange, including referrals to drug treatment and counseling.

Few needle-exchange programs exist in the United States because many state laws prohibit the possession, distribution, or sale of clean syringes. Most of these laws were designed to reduce illicit drug use. But more than one hundred needle-exchange programs exist in forty communities in twenty-eight states, resulting from a variety of legal loopholes, including exceptions to state laws and special health waivers.

Some people claim that needle-exchange programs worsen the damage caused by injection drug use, or that such programs send the message that "it's okay" to use illicit drugs. On the other hand, some people claim that needle-exchange programs do not increase drug use. The question they often pose to make their point: Does the availability of silverware alone cause a person to eat? Would the absence of silverware alone cause a person to stop eating?

In all likelihood, the debate between these two camps will continue. While politicians and activists bicker over the ethics of needle exchange, the message for you is clear: Don't share needles or other IV drug paraphernalia with anyone. Not sharing needles will also protect you from hepatitis B, hepatitis C, and other serious assaults to your immune system.

Finding a needle-exchange program isn't easy

Don't expect to find needle-exchange programs in the Yellow Pages. One good way to find a needle-exchange program near you is to call a free, 24-hour-a-day hotline operated by the Centers for Disease Control (CDC):

CDC HIV hotline
(800) 342-2437

The call is anonymous, meaning that you don't have to give your real name. However, be prepared to give the operator your zip code so he or she can try to locate an organization near you that offers a needle-exchange program.

Another option is to call an AIDS organization in your area. A list of organizations is available in the Resource Guide of this book. If you call, you might start by asking for basic information about HIV. Then, if you feel comfortable, ask about needle exchange programs in your area.

If you can't get new needles, clean them yourself

If you can't get new works, the next best thing you can do is clean them. Here's how to clean your needles and other paraphernalia:

Draw In

Shake Several
Times

Push Out

STEP 1:

Draw clean water all the way up into your set, shake it, and squirt it out. Repeat that process three times.

STEP 2:

Then do it twice with full-strength household bleach (not diluted). Try to leave the bleach in for two minutes each time.

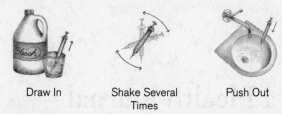

Draw In   Shake Several   Push Out
Times

STEP 3:

Finally, flush again, three times, with clean water. Clean the cooker by rinsing well with bleach, and never reuse cotton.

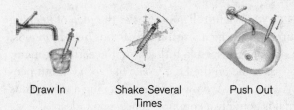

Draw In   Shake Several   Push Out
Times

IN A SENTENCE:

> *If you use needles for any reason, don't share them—get clean ones if possible or clean them yourself.*

living

Why a Health Journal Matters

AT FIRST, you might roll your eyes at the idea of keeping a health journal. Keeping a written log of your health, moods, and medications might seem a little corny, too earthy-crunchy, or "woo-woo" as some on the East Coast like to say about people on the West Coast. Woo-woo or not, keeping a meticulous health journal is actually a common-sense, good idea.

HIV is a complicated disease that slowly affects the immune system over a period of years. At the same time, healthcare in general has become increasingly complex. Your doctor or healthcare provider may not remember every detail of your situation. Furthermore, your primary-care physician might refer you to a specialist, such as a skin doctor or an ear, nose, and throat specialist. Keeping a health journal can help you keep track of important blood results that might be handy for specialists.

More than just being handy, a health journal may be what you need to keep from becoming a hypochondriac. Having HIV can make anyone wonder about a simple sniffle or itch. However, **hypochondria** is preoccupation with physical health to the point of obsession. This preoccupation with symptoms is unpleasant and can interfere with daily life in a negative way.

Keeping a health journal can be as complicated or as simple as you want to make it. If you're the kind of person who doesn't like to remember details, then a health journal is even more important. Say, for example, you have a doctor's appointment in two months. Before the visit, you might experience a minor symptom, such as swollen lymph nodes or mild fevers. If you write down your specific symptoms and the dates they occurred, then on your next visit to the doctor you can communicate the symptoms in detail to your doctor with accuracy.

A health journal should reflect the priorities that are important for you. You might want to track how often you exercise or how nutritiously you have been eating. You might be concerned about overindulging in, say, alcohol. You can write down the amount you drink over the course of weeks and months. Reading over your entries at a later time might give you a new perspective on things. Obviously, there's no limit on the details you can track with a journal, but here are a few areas you should consider tracking:

- nutrition/exercise
- key blood tests and results
- previous vaccinations and when they occurred
- your moods or negative thinking
- medications that you take and side effects
- longer-term side effects that can be caused by HIV medicine
- priorities or goals

Nutrition/exercise

Say, for example, you experience recurrent bouts of diarrhea. In this case, you might consider keeping detailed records of all the foods you eat and how they affect you. You might start by recording the time of each meal, what you eat, and how you feel afterward. Make sure that you note every significant symptom or response as it occurs.

Perhaps you decide to embark on an exercise program with a goal of a 45-minute workout three times a week. Over the course of weeks, by tracking your progress in a health journal, you can see your progress over time. You might want to keep track of weights lifted, minutes of cardio, or even exercises that you like versus ones that you dislike. Many people keep food diaries to help control their weight.

Key blood tests

As you'll learn in later chapters, there are some important blood tests for people with HIV to keep track of over time. These results will help you and your doctor assess the strength of your immune system. If, down the road, you change doctors or visit a specialist who might not have your medical records on hand, your health journal can help you maximize your interaction with the specialist. Later on you will learn more about the meaning of specific blood tests, but for now a few critical ones are:

- **CD4+ T-cell counts**: More commonly called T-cells.
- **HIV viral load**: Measures the amount of the virus in your blood.
- **Weight/body mass index**: Can help you see whether you're gaining or losing weight over time.
- **Cholesterol/triglycerides**: These tests measure the amount of special fatty substances floating around in your blood.
- **Liver tests (AST):** These tests measure the health of your liver, and for people who have underlying liver conditions, tracking the health of your liver can help them spot a problem before it gets out of hand.
- **Herpes outbreaks:** If you get cold sores or suspect you may have a form of the herpes virus, it's wise to record where on your body outbreaks occur and how often.

Vaccination schedules

It's not unusual for people to get the vaccines they need from various health-care providers over the course of their lifetimes. For example, you might have gotten one vaccine from your doctor, and then be vaccinated for something else at a community clinic or hospital. Or, you may change health-care providers as a result of moving from one region to another. You may not have a central record of your vaccines. This can create problems. For example, two important vaccines for people with HIV are the hepatitis A and hepatitis B vaccines. To make things more complicated, sometimes vaccines must be administered multiple times over the course of months. Keeping vaccination details in a health journal can help take the guesswork out of the process.

Moods shifts and negative thinking

Your moods can change over time. Testing positive for HIV might be something that triggers depression or anxiety in the months that follow. Tracking your general moods over time can be a great tool for monitoring the "health of your head." Sometimes, people who get depressed are not aware of their shifting moods. One day you might feel fine, then suddenly you're feeling sad, anxious, or angry, without knowing why. Mood changes like these may be caused by an "unfelt feeling," which might be traced to an external event. Writing down your moods and perhaps some external events can help you become more aware of your feelings and the things that upset you.

Medications and side effects

Even if you're not taking HIV medications right now, tracking what drugs you do take—and the side effects they cause—might help you sometime in the future. For example, if your doctor prescribed you an antidepressant, you can write down any side effects the drug is causing you. At your next doctor's visit, you can bring the journal and describe in detail the side effects. This way, your doctor or healthcare provider might be less likely to dismiss the symptoms as "in your head" and not worth worrying about. In fact, this works even for medications such as common antibiotics. From keeping a health journal, I've determined that an antibiotic called amoxicillin makes me queasy. Now, if my doctor asks if I am allergic to any antibiotics, I'm able to say "no, but amoxicillin makes me sick."

Long-term side effects

Some HIV medicines can cause certain side effects that can affect the general distribution of fat in your body. It's especially frustrating because these side effects are very subtle and occur slowly over the course of months and years. It might be a wise idea to start with a baseline measurement of your body. You can measure the circumference of your stomach or legs, for example. Then, write the number in your health journal. Six months later, you can take your measurements again and compare the results to see if HIV medicine is causing you any side effects. You could even take a Polaroid picture of yourself wearing nothing but your underwear, and then compare the shape of your body to another picture as time goes on. If nothing else, this will go a long way toward easing any worries you have about these side effects.

Priorities or goals

A health journal might also be a good place to write down what's important for you in a larger sense. Obviously, what's important for one person may not be important for another. You might consider taking a few minutes to think about this question. For example, in my health journal I keep a list of general priorities in my life and I rank the importance of each. I keep the list on my refrigerator and above my desk. Whenever I wonder about a difficult or perplexing situation in life, I refer back to this list to see how consistent it is among my personal priorities. For me, they include:

○ *Health.* For me, health comes first above all else.
○ *Sanity.* This is a generic term I use to remind me about stress levels, doing things that are good for my emotional health, or even keeping substance abuse in check.
○ *Relationships.* Some people say that the quality of one's life can be measured by the quality of one's relationships with other people. This priority helps remind me to keep up with friends and family.
○ *Integrity.* Not everyone feels this way, but I find it's important to try to keep my promises and do things that I believe are right for me.
○ *The Basics.* This term describes the importance of keeping up with the basic things in life, such as paying rent on time, making sure I have car insurance when I drive, and keeping close track of my income.

Setting up a health journal is easy and inexpensive

You don't need to spend much money to create a health journal. For less than five dollars, you can find a notebook or a pad of paper at any grocery store. You might want to use a notebook that also has pockets where you can keep related articles or even miscellaneous tidbits, such as health receipts or laboratory reports. First, decide the details you want to track over time. Then, with each entry, be sure to write down the date so that you have a record of any changes. You also might want to write down any questions that you want to discuss with your doctor. Don't forget to bring the health journal with you when you visit a doctor or healthcare provider. Going through your journal is a good way to pass the time while in the waiting room.

Are you a hypochondriac?

The Whiteley Index is a widely used test to determine hypochondria. As with all tests the result must be interpreted cautiously. A high score is an indication that you could profit from talking this over with your doctor. Below

Bob's Health Journal

THERE ARE many ways to use a journal and everyone is different. Here is one example of a health journal that will help you get started keeping your own journal.

NOVEMBER 19, 2007
VISITED DOCTOR ON NOVEMBER 18

doctor visit	May 2	July 12	September 7	November 18
t-cells	376	358	369	320
viral load	12,000	15,400	15,100	17,500
liver count (AST)	42	38	?	32
blood pressure	140/70	132/80	?	140/75
cholesterol	204	195	197	?
weight	?	205	204	204
symptoms	none	diarrhea	none	none
mood	depressed	okay	depressed	feel fine
general concerns	wondering when to start HIV treatment	doc says minor drop in t-cells is not a big deal for now	my t-cells are up so I feel good	doc says my rising viral load may be reason to consider HIV treatment soon

NOTE: don't worry if you miss some details in one or two visits. The important thing about a health journal is to track the details over the course of months, so you can better see the big picture and the trends over time.

is a list of questions about your health. For each one, circle the number indicating how much this is true for you.

1 = Not at all
2 = A little bit
3 = Moderately
4 = Quite a bit
5 = A great deal

1: *Do you worry a lot about your health?*
   1   2   3   4   5

2: *Do you think there is something seriously wrong with your body?*
   1   2   3   4   5

3: *Is it hard for you to forget about yourself and think about all sorts of other things?*
   1   2   3   4   5

4: *If you feel ill and someone tells you that you are looking better, do you become annoyed?*
   1   2   3   4   5

5: *Do you find that you are often aware of various things happening in your body?*
   1   2   3   4   5

6: *Are you bothered by many aches and pains?*
   1   2   3   4   5

7: *Are you afraid of illness?*
   1   2   3   4   5

8: *Do you worry about your health more than most people?*
   1   2   3   4   5

9: *Do you get the feeling that people are not taking your illnesses seriously enough?*
   1   2   3   4   5

10: *Is it hard for you to believe the doctor when he/she tells you there is nothing for you to worry about?*
   1   2   3   4   5

11: *Do you often worry about the possibility that you have a serious illness?*
1   2   3   4   5

12: *If a disease is brought to your attention (through the radio, TV, newspapers, or someone you know), do you worry about getting it yourself?*
1   2   3   4   5

13: *Do you find that you are bothered by many different symptoms?*
1   2   3   4   5

14: *Do you often have the symptoms of a very serious disease?*
1   2   3   4   5

Now add the number from all the questions above. The higher the score, the more hypochondriacal you are likely to be. There is no set cutoff score, but healthy people without anxiety generally have a score between 14 and 28. Patients with hypochondria are found to have a score between 32 and 55. These numbers are merely indications to help you find out if you have hypochondria. A high score may also signal symptoms of depression or anxiety disorders.

IN A SENTENCE:

When you're newly diagnosed with HIV, keeping a health journal can help you see the big picture and may help keep you from worrying about minor or normal symptoms.

learning

Take Your Time to Adjust

MOST PEOPLE don't need to start HIV medicine immediately. HIV affects individuals differently. It's important for you
to find out the health of your immune system. A doctor will
draw some samples of blood and you'll get at least two test
results. Depending on the results, you'll either start taking HIV
medicine or you won't.

The decision to begin or delay HIV medicine is your own.
Nobody can force you to start. Even if your immune system is
severely damaged, you can take certain medications to prevent
specific diseases, which may buy you more time to think about
your options.

You have time to make your own decisions. Don't let yourself
be pressured into starting treatment, or a particular kind of
treatment. Take things slowly, talk to your doctor or other experienced people. Only rarely does the decision need to be made
in a hurry. Usually there's a lot of time to consider all the
options.

Don't let the details overwhelm you

You might feel as if there's a lot of information coming at you
right now. What's worth knowing? For right now, focus on the
likelihood and the *severity* of potential health issues. For example: how *likely* is it that you get an AIDS-related condition? And
if you do get an AIDS-related condition, how *severe* could it be?

For example, coming down with full-blown AIDS is bad. However, if your immune system is strong, it's unlikely to happen to you in the next three years. Exactly how long you have depends on how strong your immune system is.

Out of one hundred people with HIV who have strong immune systems, about fifteen will come down with AIDS within the next three years. Among people whose immune systems are damaged, the risk doubles to thirty in one hundred, or 30 percent.

This is a number that you can trust. Researchers have studied thousands of people with HIV. They find a predictable percentage of people get sick over time. Your chances of getting sick relate directly to the strength of your immune system.

What does a 30 percent chance look like?

IMAGINE THAT the diagram below is a target in a game of darts. Throw the dart once and your chance of hitting the gray zone is 30 percent. If one hundred people throw the dart, about thirty people will hit the gray zone.

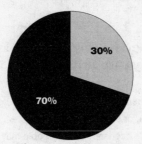

Simply having HIV puts you at a higher risk for getting sick or dying compared to people without the virus. As your immune system becomes more damaged, your risk of getting sick becomes greater. However, you can improve your odds with HIV treatment, which halts the damage to your immune system by stopping the virus. With less virus in your body, your immune system can rebuild itself.

Adjust to the news first before telling others

Early on, consider keeping the news to a select few until you get a better handle on what's happening for yourself. Telling family members, co-workers, even some friends might create more problems than it's worth.

The best person to confide in may not be the person who is closest to you. If you have a tight-knit family or social group, or you live in a small community or a rural town, confidentiality is harder to maintain. Consider discussing your diagnosis with people outside of these situations, such as a counselor or trusted friend in another town or city.

Unfortunately, HIV remains a stigma for families and in the workplace. Some people have family members with a lot of their own problems," says Daniel S. Berger, M.D., medical director of Northstar Medical Center.

"Also, I think people should not be open about their HIV status in the workplace because other people will be making decisions against them, based on that knowledge. Unfortunately, that's still the reality."

Ultimately, you don't have to tell anyone about your HIV status. This includes family, friends, employers, coworkers, or health-care providers. Unless there's a compelling reason—like you're a surgeon or a prize-fighter—there's no reason why you should tell anyone at work. If you need to leave work early for a doctor's appointment, leave it at that. Otherwise, you risk potentially serious and unnecessary discrimination and disruption.

On the other hand, if telling someone will truly make things easier for you, then the benefits might outweigh the consequences. But before you disclose the news, think about it carefully.

Quick considerations about disclosing your HIV status to others:

- Be clear with yourself about why you want to tell this person. Do you want sympathy, special treatment, or support?
- Consider the worst-case scenario. Some people may become hysterical. Are you able to deal with that?
- Give people plenty of time to process the information. Things might seem fine at first, but this can change down the road.
- Think carefully before telling a spouse or partner right off the bat. It will raise enormous issues for them. Choose a setting that offers you plenty of time and privacy.

Calling hotlines is one way to practice talking about HIV

When it comes to HIV, some people prefer to talk to someone anonymously. "People don't just have HIV issues, they often have issues with their sexual orientation, lifestyles, or substance abuse," says Rossetta M., who also works as a health educator. "People need to be hooked up with people who parallel them and who have been successful with HIV."

Many AIDS organizations around the county offer hotlines, counseling services, and even "HIV buddy" programs. You can find a list of local AIDS organizations in the Resource Guide at the back of this book.

In most cases, people with HIV have plenty of time to adjust to the news. There's no rush; you're not going anywhere soon. You can postpone telling people for days, months, or even years.

When considering whom to tell, take your time. Think about the consequences carefully. Don't tell too many people in the beginning, before you've had a chance to process things for yourself. If possible, you might consider talking with an HIV-positive person first. This way, you can practice what you will say.

Did you know?

○ There are laws designed to protect people with HIV against discrimination in health, employment, housing, and education situations.
○ You do not have to tell your employer that you have HIV.
○ Health professionals are not supposed to treat you differently because of your HIV status.

IN A SENTENCE:

Adjusting to life with HIV takes time, so relax, don't let the details overwhelm you, and selectively talk with other people.

FIRST-WEEK MILESTONE

By the end of the first week, you've come a long way in understanding and accepting your HIV diagnosis.

- ○ YOU KNOW THAT TODAY HIV IS A MANAGEABLE CHRONIC DISEASE, AND, BY TAKING CONTROL OF YOUR HEALTH, YOU CAN EXPECT TO HAVE A FULL LIFE AND LIVE TO A NORMAL LIFE EXPECTANCY.

- ○ YOU KNOW TO EXPECT A VARIETY OF DIFFICULT EMOTIONS INCLUDING SHOCK, SADNESS, ANXIETY, FEELING "SEPARATE FROM YOURSELF," SELF-BLAME, ANGER, AND DENIAL—ALL OF WHICH ARE NORMAL REACTIONS.

- ○ YOU RECOGNIZE THAT BEING HEALTHY REQUIRES MAKING HEALTHY CHOICES IN LIFE.

- ○ YOU UNDERSTAND THAT HIV STIGMA IS COMMON IN SOCIETY AND MAY LEAD TO PERSONAL FEELINGS OF SHAME.

- ○ YOU KNOW THAT TALKING TO OTHER PEOPLE WITH HIV CAN HELP YOU BETTER DEAL WITH YOUR OWN SITUATION.

Finding the Best HIV Doctor

THERE'S A LOT on your mind now. The last thing you probably want to think about is your doctor. The good news is that once you get a good doctor, you can worry a lot less. Maybe you already have a primary physician. Regardless, now is a good time to consider—or reconsider—the person who will guide your HIV care in the future.

Smart patients find smart doctors

Doctors are a little like mechanics. Most people visit a mechanic when something goes wrong with a car. Most people visit a doctor only when they're sick. But the parallel doesn't end there. If you've ever had car troubles, you probably compare your options or shop around, at least a little. Now that you have HIV, it's important that you understand that having a good HIV doctor will help you live longer. Studies have shown this to be true. Think about it: Do you treat yourself as well as you would treat your car?

The number-one advice that Anthony S. Fauci, M.D., director of the National Institute of Allergy and Infectious Diseases, offers people with HIV is to find a trusted physician or health-care provider. "Get a physician whom you trust, who's knowledgeable, and who has experience," says Fauci, "and don't hesitate to get a second opinion."

Patient advocates are pushing these days to make HIV treatment a medical specialty with its own training and certification, similar to cancer treatment or diabetes treatment. Advocates say that doctors who don't specialize in HIV are less likely to keep up with fast-changing drug therapies and treatment strategies.

On the other hand, a doctor who focuses only on HIV may overlook the bigger picture. "There are some good points about specific credentialing for HIV because you intensify the knowledge in a particular area," says Fauci. "But I'm afraid if you get too narrow, you're going to wind up keeping out some of the other specialties that you really need to be involved in the total care of an individual with HIV.

"People with HIV need to start thinking not just in terms of HIV—but of the totality of health. You are treating the whole person. You're not just treating a virus anymore. The whole person has lots of other things going on.

"My recommendation for physicians who are going to be—and are— taking care of people with HIV is that it's no longer appropriate to just be an HIV expert," says Fauci. "If you're an HIV expert, you have to be an expert in all the other things that beset a person with HIV."

Find an HIV specialist with diverse training— and whom you like

People have different philosophies when it comes to their doctors. Some people prefer a more aggressive doctor, while others feel more comfortable with a gentler bedside manner. There are trade-offs to each.

The aggressive doctor may be more up-to-date on new HIV research. He or she may even attend HIV conferences or be involved in cutting-edge research studies. HIV treatment changes all the time, so this type of doctor may be able to offer more options. The downside, however, is usually that the aggressive doctor may spend less time with you and your situation.

The warmer and fuzzier HIV doctor may have a better bedside manner. He or she may pay more attention to you, your symptoms, and your worries. This type of doctor may ask about your life in general and how you're feeling overall. In general, this type of physician may be less informed about new medical information or strategies.

Doctors are as different as auto mechanics. If you don't like the guy who changes your oil, you get a new one, right? Finding or changing doctors is obviously not as simple, but that's the idea. Ultimately, the relationship between you and your doctor is a transaction between two people. You get something from your doctor and your doctor gets something from you.

Here's a list of what you should look for when searching for an HIV doctor:

- **Medical training.** Find a physician who is board certified in internal medicine, infectious diseases, or a related specialty. One good suggestion is to phone the potential doctor's receptionist and ask about the doctor's credentials.

- **Experience working with people with HIV.** Some physicians, particularly in New York, Los Angeles, Miami, and other metropolitan areas, devote most of their practices to treating people with HIV. A doctor who is knowledgeable about HIV will be able to offer you more information and options. Does the doctor belong to the Infectious Disease Society of America or other professional groups involved in AIDS treatment? (If a doctor evades the question, that ought to tell you something.)

- **Similar philosophies and attitudes.** Some doctors follow a conservative, safe, by-the-book approach to medicine. Others are more willing to try new or alternative therapies. Consider your own philosophies first so you'll know what to look for in a doctor.

- **Receptiveness to your input.** Will your doctor listen to your suggestions, complaints, or feelings? If you bring information, will he or she read it and respond?

- **Availability.** Consider the average waiting time for office visits, particularly on your initial visit. Also, think about how quickly your doctor returns phone calls or e-mails. But remember, most doctors are overwhelmed with patients and work. After your first visit, expect to get about fifteen minutes of your doctor's time per visit. (Later in this chapter, you'll learn how to make the most of those minutes).

- **Affordability.** Unless you can afford to pay upfront for your medical services, it's likely that your choices will be dictated by the type of healthcare coverage you have. If you have Medicaid, you'll need to find a doctor or clinic that accepts it. If you don't have health insurance, your choices may be even more limited. Call ahead and ask about payment and billing procedures. Work out an acceptable financial arrangement in advance. Remember, you will be monitoring your HIV for years. Medical bills have a way of stacking up faster than you might think, and in ways you might not expect. Large medical bills can become a problem down the road.

○ **Level of comfort.** You will need to be honest about your lifestyle with your doctor. Your sexual practices and use of recreational drugs will eventually surface as a topic of discussion. If your doctor seems too judgmental, keep searching. It's better to have a doctor who really knows you.

○ **Follow your intuition.** If you don't like the way a potential doctor runs his practice, continue searching. In the long run, it's better to take some time to find the right doctor than it is to change doctors down the road.

○ **Confidentiality.** Some people are very concerned about keeping their HIV status private. You might choose to get your HIV care from a provider in another town to protect your privacy. You will need to find your own balance between confidentiality and convenience.

A good HIV doctor is hard to find

Not sure exactly how to go about finding a good HIV doctor who's right for you? Below is a plan of action for you. It's one way to organize the process of doctor hunting, which may be obvious to some, but not to others, since most people don't think much about doctors until they're sick. Either way, you will be developing a long-term relationship with your physician. The more advance planning you can do now, the better chance you'll have finding a good HIV doctor. And having a good HIV doctor can translate to living longer and better.

STEP 1
Remember that your ultimate goal is to find an HIV-smart doctor with whom you're comfortable and you can afford to see regularly. It might help to make a list of specific traits you want in your doctor. That's your goal.

STEP 2
What specific things could prevent you from finding your perfect doctor? One obstacle might be an understandable fear of discussing HIV or sexual issues with unfamiliar people. Another roadblock might be not having health insurance. Now, write down—or at least think about—anything that might block you from getting what you want in Step 1.

STEP 3

Now, pick one obstacle and creatively think about how to get around it. Write down the ways in which you imagine sidestepping all the obstacles you listed in Step 2. For example, if you're uncomfortable discussing sex or recreational drugs with your doctor, one solution might be interviewing several doctors until you come across one who seems "in tune" with those issues. Another example might be a lack of health insurance. There are plenty of ways to get insurance but it takes research and effort on your part. Or you might choose to find a public health clinic that offers HIV care. Either way, try to imagine a way to get what you want—even if you don't have the emotional courage or the money right now. Life has a funny way of changing for the better, if you're receptive.

STEP 4

Call several local AIDS organizations and ask them for physician referrals. There's a list of AIDS organizations in the Resources section at the end of this book. In most cases, the organization will only give you a list of doctors, their names, numbers, and addresses, nothing else. The organization may not want to favor one doctor over another. Make a list of five or six potential doctors.

STEP 5

If you have any friends with HIV, ask if they are familiar with the doctors on your list. Also, ask them for recommendations and find out how they selected their HIV physician. If you don't know anyone with HIV or don't want to discuss the subject, go online or try calling the doctor's office to see what you can uncover. Remember to ask specifically about insurance and billing procedures. This will help you narrow your list to maybe two or three.

STEP 6

Make an appointment with your top choice, but commit yourself to interviewing at least one other doctor. This way, you'll be able to compare the two. Make clear that you just want to get to know the doctor. Most doctors' offices are—or should be, anyway—receptive to this request. Sometimes these initial consultations are free, but not always. You'll know it when you find the right doctor.

Your doctor is not your friend

Once you've decided on a doctor, schedule an initial visit. Remember, your doctor is not your friend; he's your doctor. There's a lot of talk these days about developing a "doctor-patient relationship." This concept is great in theory, but in reality, the relationship is a transaction. Your doctor is getting paid, either by you, your insurance company, or the government, to keep you healthy.

There's a myth about "special relationships" between doctors and patients. However, competition for shrinking healthcare dollars, the growing numbers of health maintenance organizations (HMOs), and the push toward the "managed care" model of practice have long ago smashed this myth. "Managed care" refers to a variety of techniques for influencing healthcare providers and/or patients. The overall aim of managed care is to contain the cost, the quality, or the access to certain expensive health services.

In fact, some forms of managed care offer a financial incentive for doctors to spend less time with each patient. For instance, some preferred provider organizations (PPOs) may pay less to doctors per patient, but will promise them more patients instead. What this means to you is less time to talk to your doctor.

According to surveys published in the *New England Journal of Medicine*, American physicians spend an average of eighteen to twenty minutes with each patient. My experience of seeing HIV doctors on a regular basis is that, after the initial visit, you're lucky if you get fifteen minutes. But it's not necessarily a bad thing; it's just a reality to which you'll need to adjust.

Making the most of your fifteen minutes requires advanced planning on your part. At some point before your appointment, make a list of topics to discuss. Keep the list in your pocket and carry a pen or pencil with you during the visit. Check off the items on your list as your doctor addresses them. You may feel weird or awkward about this at first, but your doctor will soon learn that you mean business. He or she will likely perceive you as a more organized, directed patient and, therefore, will be more likely to address all of your concerns. Try this just once with your doctor and you'll notice the difference.

Expect to talk a lot during the initial visit

So that you know what to expect from your first official visit, be prepared to discuss:

○ **Your health history.** Your doctor will ask when you first tested positive for HIV and if you have any symptoms, such as fevers, night sweats, weight loss, diarrhea, skin rashes, or changes in your mental status. Be prepared for questions about sexually transmitted diseases, chicken pox or shingles, viral hepatitis, bacterial infections, gyneco-logic problems, and exposure to tuberculosis (TB), and where you've lived or traveled.

○ **Sexual practices**. You will be asked about behaviors that might lead to further transmission of HIV. Your doctor will probably want to know if your sexual partners are aware of your HIV status. You'll probably be encouraged to inform your partners of your HIV status. You are also likely to get a lesson on condoms and safer sex practices.

○ **Recreational substances and/or injecting drugs**. You may be asked about how much alcohol you drink, if you smoke marijuana, or use "party" drugs. If a doctor suspects you inject drugs, you'll probably be asked about your drug-using practices, your source of needles, whether you share needles, and if so, with whom.

○ **Depression.** Depression is common in people with HIV. Your doc-tor may ask about changes in mood, libido, sleeping patterns, appetite, concentration, and memory. Also, your doctor will proba-bly ask whom you have informed of your HIV status and what kinds of support you have. This discussion may include questions about partners, children, family, living situations, and work environments.

Expect a little touching during the physical exam

During a first visit, you should expect a complete physical examination. Your doctor should look at your skin and inside your mouth, feel your lymph nodes and certain areas near your stomach, and listen to your lungs as you breathe in and out. Your doctor might even want to examine your anus, penis, or vagina.

First-visit checklist

A good HIV doctor should perform a number of tests on you. But depending on your situation, you may not have access to a good HIV doc-tor. Just in case, here's a list of the most important tests you should ask about on your first visit:

○ **Repeat HIV test.** If you were tested anonymously or don't have documentation of your HIV status, your doctor might repeat the HIV test. HIV tests are extremely accurate but false positives can occur from clerical errors.

- ○ **HIV viral load.** This test measures the amount of the virus in your blood (further chapters discuss this topic in more detail).
- ○ **T-Cell (CD4+) counts.** This gauges the status of your immune system (further chapters discuss this topic in more detail).
- ○ **Complete blood count.** This test examines different aspects of your blood.
- ○ **Syphilis test.** It's possible to have this sexually transmitted disease and not know it.
- ○ **TB testing.** It's also possible to have been exposed to TB and not know it.
- ○ **Toxoplasmosis testing.** This is a common infection that people can get through raw meat or handling cat litter.
- ○ **Viral hepatitis.** You and your doctor will want to know if you have been exposed to hepatitis A, hepatitis B, and/or hepatitis C.
- ○ **Gynecological tests.** Women with HIV are at increased risk for a number of gynecological problems. Make sure you get a pelvic examination with Pap smear.
- ○ **Other lab tests**. Depending on your age, sex, and other variables, there may be further tests your doctor will want. Consider an anal Pap smear for men and women.
- ○ **Vaccines.** There are a number of important vaccines that you can ask about. They include:
  - ○ pneumonia
  - ○ hepatitis A
  - ○ hepatitis B
  - ○ dT (tetanus booster)
  - ○ influenza vaccine
  - ○ HPV

IN A SENTENCE:

Shop around before choosing an HIV doctor, and make the most of your limited time with that person.

learning

The Virus Versus You

MOST PEOPLE think viruses are creepy. You hear about this virus or that virus and rarely are they good news. So why bother to read more about HIV? If your goal is to live longer and better—and you're facing a medical challenge—you should ask a lot of questions, especially of your doctor.

You'll pose better questions and you'll get better answers if you appear to have a good medical vocabulary. But don't worry too much if you don't understand all the words and phrases associated with HIV right now.

However, if you're anything like me, words like **pathogenesis** make me want to run. When I start reading technical literature, I always manage to find distractions like cleaning my room or chasing flies with the DustBuster.

Here's a brief look at how the Human Immunodeficiency Virus (HIV) works.

HIV is a little like a terrorist

The drama begins when HIV somehow finds its way into the bloodstream, where it floats around for a while undetected. At first, you might think HIV is a smart virus. To the contrary, it's actually dumb compared to other viruses. What HIV has on its side is luck. It's a lucky virus because it always manages to find what it needs to survive.

In the bloodstream, the invader eventually sets off an alarm. This alarm, in a simple sense, is the creation of antibodies. Think of antibodies as similar to early-warning sentinels who scour the countryside looking for potential troublemakers. When an antibody sees trouble, it reports it back to immune central. And it always remembers the bad guys.

With the antibody alarm tripped, the immune system is made aware of an illegal break-in. Think of your body as a country or nation. In this analogy, the human immune system is like a country's department of defense. The immune system defends your body from attack.

This immune defense responds by sending out an army of white blood cells, also known as **T-cells.** Ordinarily, T-cells are excellent soldiers. They're a critical part of the body's first and most robust response to foreign invasion. Different T-cells have different skills, but working together, the army is almost always successful.

One important and unique type of T-cell is called the **CD4 cell**. It makes up the bulk of the body's immune defenses. As fate would have it, HIV prefers to infect CD4 cells—the very cell designed to defeat foreign invaders. In fact, the virus easily enters the CD4 cell and actually uses it as a hideout and a place to grow.

Hiding inside the CD4, HIV then hijacks the cell's DNA factory. The virus uses the cell's own DNA to produce replicas of itself. Imagine if a foreign invader took control of a country's own bullet factory to make more bullets! Not bad for a dumb virus.

With a lot more replicas of itself, HIV bursts out of the T-cell factory, looking for more conquests. Eventually, the T-cell dies. Generally speaking, this process takes about two and a half days.

HIV is fortunate in that it multiples in great numbers. Within twenty-four hours, HIV reproduces itself about ten billion times—roughly equivalent to creating twice the number of all humans on the earth each and every day. Compared with other viruses, HIV's replication rate is high. This gives it a distinct advantage called "resistance," as you'll learn in later chapters.

Size up your enemy by measuring your viral load

The amount of virus swimming in the bloodstream is called the viral level or, more commonly, **viral load**. A high viral load means there's a lot of HIV in the blood. An undetectable viral load is a good thing, because it means there's very little virus in the blood. An undetectable viral load does not mean you can't give the virus to someone else.

In general, the viral load test measures how fast HIV disease is progressing. If someone has a high viral load, HIV is very active, and vice versa. On the other hand, the CD4 cell count reflects how far HIV disease has progressed. In general:

A good thing
  High T-cell counts (not very far)
  Low or undetectable viral loads (not very fast)
A bad thing
  Low T-cell counts (progressed far)
  High viral load (progressing fast)

There's a war between your immune system and HIV

There's an ongoing war between HIV and the immune system. During the course of infection, however, this balance of power shifts from side to side. During the first few days of infection, HIV gets the upper hand. This is called acute infection. During an acute infection with HIV, many people report symptoms similar to those with flu.

Once the immune department gets busy, the balance of power is restored. Within months of acute infection, the amount of HIV in the blood is generally reduced and the immune system holds back the virus. This extraordinary balance of power can go on for years.

At some point, however, the immune system begins to run short on soldiers. This leaves HIV with the ability to replicate uncontrollably and to ultimately destroy any remaining T-cells. Without disease-fighting T-cells, the human body is fair game for a host of other unfriendly invaders, ranging from irritating to life-threatening.

By the way, the above process of how HIV does damage is called *pathogenesis*. There, that wasn't so bad.

Call in your secret weapons when you need help

Antivirals are chemical compounds that, for one reason or another, can interfere with viruses. Specifically HIV is a type of virus called a **retrovirus**. As such, chemical compounds that work against HIV are **antiretrovirals**. I find that word intimidating and hard to read, so I'll just continue using "antiviral" to describe a chemical that slows HIV.

Remember the analogy of the immune system being the department of defense? In this case, antivirals would be like spies. At any point in the conflict between the immune system and HIV, the antiviral spies can be called in. However, the spies don't answer to your immune system, they answer only to you. You decide when the time is right.

Different antivirals are designed to accomplish different tasks. Some antivirals infiltrate the DNA factory and render it useless. Hence the virus can no longer make copies of itself. Other antivirals prevent the final assembly of newly manufactured particles of virus. A more detailed discussion of the antiviral classes will come later. For now, I'll just introduce you to the major players on the antiviral block:

○ nucleosides (or nukes)
○ non-nucleosides (or non-nukes)
○ protease inhibitors (pronounced *pro-tee-aze*)

The best way to use these drugs is to combine them in different ways. This is called **combination therapy,** and you've probably heard it referred to as the "**AIDS cocktail**." Another name is **highly active antiretroviral therapy (HAART)**. The term *HAART* first cropped up in HIV lingo because some drug combinations were not considered "highly active." Today, the antivirals and the combinations are vastly improved.

IN A SENTENCE:

> Armed with a good HIV specialist and a basic understanding of how HIV operates, you're on the road to making better choices for a healthier and happier life.

Before You Disclose Your HIV Status to Anyone

IT'S EASY to imagine a time when HIV test results will be delivered over the Internet. Today, some people get their results by U.S. mail or telephone. No matter how you received your HIV diagnosis, eventually you'll find yourself having a conversation about HIV with someone else.

The thought of disclosing your HIV status to certain people in your life may make you nervous. The good news is that you don't have to tell everyone. You can be selective about whom you tell.

When you're ready, you'll want to think about deciding whom to tell and whom not to tell. Of course, there's no rule about this because it will change for you over time. This week, you might tell a trusted friend. Next month, you might tell strangers in a support group. Down the road, you may tell your parents or your children. Or you might choose never to tell anyone.

The decision to disclose your HIV status to others is always and only yours. However, everyone has their opinion on the subject. Some groups claim the only deciding factor in telling other people is whether or not other people come in direct contact with your bodily fluids such as blood, semen, or vaginal secretions. Others say it's good to tell friends or family for support.

Whatever people say, the reality is that people with HIV are selective about disclosing their health status. According to one study, the process of choosing which individuals to tell the news often involves anguish and uncertainty. Another study found that HIV-positive people were often indecisive about disclosing their HIV status.

How we feel about disclosing our HIV status

- ○ 40 percent report indecision about HIV disclosure
- ○ 31 percent planned never to tell certain people
- ○ 28 percent desired to reveal their status to someone
- ○ 21 percent regretted having told someone

Why disclose your HIV status?

The reasons to disclose one's HIV status will be different for everyone. Whatever your specific reason for wanting to tell someone, chances are good it will fall in one of several general categories. They include:

- ○ the "right" for others to know
- ○ need for emotional support from others
- ○ access to medical resources or services
- ○ the need for intimacy
- ○ integrity

There are pros and cons to disclosing your HIV status

Who should you tell that you're HIV-positive? The answer to this question depends on what you want from the person whom you're thinking about telling. You might tell a spouse or partner for emotional support or for his or her own health. You might decide not to tell your children because they're not old enough to grasp "adult" ideas.

Think carefully about whom you tell. As it turns out, about one in five people regret telling their HIV status to someone. The following are some risks and benefits to disclosing your HIV status:

SPOUSE/PARTNER

Potential Benefits: If you have a husband, wife, boyfriend, girlfriend, long-term partner, or whatever you call it, you may find comfort in the support that person can offer. Perhaps your other half can do some of the chores around the house. Maybe they can listen to your worries and give suggestions. Maybe they can pick you up from the doctor's visit. Maybe they'll just listen to your feelings.

Potential Risks: It's possible that your partner may become alarmed by his or her own HIV status. Instead of being supportive, your primary partner may feel nervous about himself or herself. If the two of you aren't getting along these days, an HIV-positive diagnosis in one or both of you is likely to further strain the relationship. Of course, this isn't a suggestion to avoid a rocky relationship by keeping secrets, but if your love life is already on the rocks, consider the timing of telling your partner. You need to cope with the news first. A little "time away" for you to get your own head together might be appropriate.

FRIENDS

Potential Benefits: Studies show that most people disclose their HIV diagnosis to close friends or current partners within days of first learning the news themselves. A close friend may be able to offer new ways of thinking about your situation. He or she may be the best form of support for you by simply listening to you.

Potential Risks: Some people are more informed about HIV than others. A friend may appear comfortable with the news at first, but may turn out to be uncomfortable with that news in the long run. There's no shortage of stories about "friends" disappearing after learning of one's HIV status.

DOCTORS AND DENTISTS

Potential Benefits: Disclosing your HIV status to an HIV doctor should be easy enough. However, people often encounter different types of doctors. While there's reason to tell your primary-care physician, there's no reason why your foot doctor needs to know. Dentists are a different story. In theory, your dentist should be using what are called "universal precautions," which are special procedures to avoid any kind of virus, not just HIV. While you're not legally bound to disclose to your dentist, he or she may be able to help identify certain health problems.

Potential Risks: As with counselors, some doctors may be required by law to report certain events. The regulations vary among states, cities, hospitals, HMOs, and individual practices. By telling a doctor, you risk losing a degree of privacy. As for some nurses and other healthcare workers, like it or not they might be uncomfortable working with someone who they think has HIV.

THERAPISTS AND PSYCHOLOGISTS

Potential Benefits: The benefits of talking to a therapist, social worker, psychologist, or psychiatrist about HIV can be immense. You will probably find comfort in having an objective person to talk with about any number of personal issues that you may be confronting. Some of these issues may include substance abuse, sexual identity, pregnancy, and relationships. My experience has been generally good in terms of disclosing my HIV status to therapists and psychologists. In fact, an experienced social worker or therapist is very likely to offer the best support for you right now.

Potential Risks: If a social worker, therapist, or "shrink" lacks experience with HIV and related issues, you might find the opposite of comfort. It's possible he or she might guide you in a direction that is not productive for you now. You may not be emotionally ready to deal with certain topics. You may disagree about sexuality, religion, spirituality, or morality. These disagreements may cause unnecessary conflict for you at the moment and you'll end up avoiding therapy altogether. If you find yourself too uncomfortable, or even offended for some reason, speak up and terminate the relationship.

SEX PARTNERS AND ONE-NIGHT STANDS

Potential Benefits: The case for disclosing your HIV status to a potential sex partner or one-night stand has little to do with the other person. It's about you and how you conduct yourself in life. Of course, conventional wisdom holds that people with HIV are supposed to inform other people before having sex with them. Besides social and peer pressure to disclose, some state laws actually make it a crime not to disclose.

But laws that attempt to control sexual behavior usually have other motives than protection of public health. If you're having safe sex with other people, the risk to them is low, so there's no moral imperative to uphold. Besides, what matters morally—ultimately—is what you do sexually, not what you say. The real benefit of disclosing to sex partners comes from having the strength of character to be honest in difficult circumstances. Going through life being ashamed about certain aspects of your life has a way of making those aspects truly shameful.

Potential Risks: Telling people you have HIV before having sex with them almost always changes the way people behave sexually. You're more than likely to encounter some negative response, if not outright rejection. They may become afraid to have sex or even to kiss. Although a lot of people these days know about safe sex and how the virus is transmitted, there's still a great deal of stigma and fear. Even if you try to educate people about the topic, their emotions may be too strong. Irrational fear is a hard thing to overcome. If you're a person who gets hurt easily by rejection, you have a tough road ahead of you.

PARENTS

Potential Benefits: If your parents are living and you have a good relationship with one or both of them, your disclosure about being HIV-positive may lead to a stronger relationship in general. Think about it, if you had a child who tested HIV-positive, would you want to know?

Potential Risks: Sometimes parents can have so much emotional investment in your well-being, the news may devastate one or both of them. You may find yourself having to educate them about HIV or provide them with emotional support—and if you're not ready for this, it may add more stress. If the relationship with your parents is less than perfect, the news will most likely worsen the relationship.

SIBLINGS AND CLOSE FAMILY MEMBERS

Potential Benefits: Statistically, family members are usually the last to be told about someone's HIV status—unless that family member is also a friend. You may have a brother, sister, uncle, aunt, or extended family member with whom you can share the news. Disclosing your HIV status may help you feel less alone. Some HIV-positive people practice telling their brothers and sisters before telling their parents.

Potential Risks: A close family member may be less educated about HIV and the ways people contract it. For example, a sister may take the news in stride until she has her first child. At which point, she may think twice about letting you play with the baby. In addition, although some confidantes may feel privileged and will offer support, others may feel burdened, such as the sibling who must now conceal your HIV status from your parents.

CO-WORKERS

Potential Benefits: You may have friends with whom you work. (I'll discuss employers later.) They might provide an opportunity for you to discuss your health concerns as they relate to your work.

Potential Risks: People love to gossip, especially about coworkers. Like it or not, it happens. You may tell a co-worker about your diagnosis in confidence, only to later find that confidence broken. Work settings are basically rumor mills. Tell the wrong person and you might as well make an announcement at the company picnic.

One man's experience:

"Mom, Dad . . . the good news is that I'm gay."

AT AN HIV support group, I met this guy named Eric. He was having a hard time telling his parents that he was HIV-positive. The primary obstacle, as he explained it, was that his parents didn't know he was gay. At the time, Eric was about twenty-four years old and had been having sexual encounters with other men for about three years. At the support group, he rehearsed what he thought the conversation might be.

He had called them in advance and told them there was something important he wanted to tell them. He had planned to spend only one afternoon at his parents' house and break the news during that time. A week later, he reported back. He had gathered his parents around the kitchen table and, after some small talk, he broke the news: "Mom, dad, the good news is that I'm gay." Before they could respond, he then declared that he was also HIV-positive. His mother broke down in tears. His father was stone cold. Eric gave his parents some articles and brochures about HIV and then left.

In the weeks that followed, the relationship between Eric and his parents was stormy. After several months, he reported that his parents eventually adjusted to the news.

IN A SENTENCE:

It's always your own choice to tell other people about your HIV status, so be selective and think carefully about the risks and benefits of disclosing.

learning

Urban Legends, Myths, and Anti-AIDS Propaganda

People are putting HIV/AIDS infected needles underneath gas pump handles, so when someone reaches to pick it up and put gas in their car, they get stabbed with the needle. Sixteen people have been a victim of this crime so far and ten tested HIV-positive. Even if you don't drive, a family member might. What if they were next?

THIS IS not a true story. It's an urban legend. No evidence exists that anything similar to this horrifying tale truly took place. Nonetheless, it was anonymously posted on the Internet in 2006 and proliferated much like a computer virus. HIV and AIDS have been the subject of countless urban legends over the last twenty-five years. One favorite of mine is:

Drug users are now taking their used needles and putting them into the coin return slots in public telephones. People are putting their fingers in to recover coins or just to check if anyone left change. They are getting stuck by these needles and infected with hepatitis, HIV, and other diseases.

For some reason, I now think twice before recovering my change from the phones at the airport. Politically correct or not,

legends and myths persist because they appeal to human nature. The value
of these so-called lessons is not in the storylines; it's in the people that read
them. Legends and myths about HIV just reflect the ways that our society
feels about HIV.

Fiction appeals to human nature

The tawdry or the terrifying has forever appealed to human nature.
So, if you come across something about HIV, consider what you think is
a fact and, conversely, what you think is someone's opinion. Most im-
portantly, consider the source. What is the motive of the source supplying
the information?

You'll encounter different kinds of information about HIV. Your doctor
may offer you advice. Maybe you will come across an informational Web
site on the Internet. Perhaps you will read an article or see an advertise-
ment in a local or community newspaper. Some of that information will be
good and some bad. Some information will apply directly to you, while
much of it won't.

Keep in mind that it's a free country. We like freedom of speech here in
the United States. Compared to citizens in other countries, we are afforded
a good deal of freedom, especially for the press. Like it or not, most everybody is allowed an opinion. Conflict happens when people express their
opinions disguised as fact. Any bozo with thirty-five dollars can create a Web
site to promote an opinion or advertise a product. But that doesn't mean you
should believe his or her claims.

Here's a checklist for assessing other people's advice, opinions, or
information:

- ○ What part of the message is true? What part actually exists?
- ○ What part of the message is someone's opinion?
- ○ What's the motive of the source?

AIDS conspiracies persist because they're good fiction

Conventional wisdom holds that HIV causes AIDS. Most people agree
this is true. It does so by depleting the immune system, which leaves the
human body vulnerable to opportunistic infections. But this wasn't always
conventional wisdom.

There was a time when researchers didn't know that HIV was responsible for AIDS. In the early 1980s, researchers suspected that a newly

discovered virus had some association with a growing number of sick people, but the suspicions were not proved scientifically until much later.

These days, there's indisputable research to say that HIV causes AIDS. Think about it: Since the introduction of HIV viral load testing and reliable antiviral drugs, the death rate from AIDS has dropped dramatically.

The 1980s and the early 1990s—before new techniques and good HIV drugs—were a grim time for people with HIV and AIDS. Out of despair, many people sought alternative viewpoints. In 1987, Professor Peter Duesberg, of the University of California, Berkeley, vocalized his suspicion that HIV was not the cause of AIDS, basically saying there wasn't sufficient evidence to make the claim.

With passing years, studies have repeatedly disproved Duesberg's claims. Today, the mainstream medical community considers him to be a crackpot at best, and a danger at worst. Nonetheless, his followers adopted Duesberg's theory. Over the years, fringe groups have grown, feeding on suspicion.

Today, the suspicion that HIV does not cause AIDS is alive and well—and more commonly referred to as the "AIDS myth." The AIDS myth is the theory that HIV is actually a harmless virus, doing nothing more than piggybacking on your body.

"Toxins" do not cause AIDS

If the AIDS myth is true, then you're stuck with the problem: What causes AIDS? Duesberg proposed a "toxicological explanation" for the epidemic. "Toxicological" was Duesberg's way of saying "poison." Over the years, Duesberg's "poison causes AIDS" theory has taken several turns. In 1997—before success with the AIDS cocktail was documented—Duesberg wrote about what he called the "drug-AIDS hypothesis." Duesberg claims that the use of recreational drugs, like cocaine, crystal, poppers, and heroin, is a cause of AIDS. Another source of AIDS, he says, is the same antiviral drugs designed to stop AIDS. The height of Duesberg's popularity was just before new HIV treatments dramatically improved treatment. And over time, Duesberg's outdated "which came first, chicken or egg?" hypothesis has been disproved again and again.

Word Games: Pick Your Poison

TOX OR TOXI — prefixes that relates to the word poison

TOXIC — describes a substance that is poisonous

TOXICITY — state of being poisonous

TOXIN — a poisonous substance made by your own body

TOXICOLOGICAL — anything related to poison

TOXICOLOGY — a science that deals with effects and problems of poison

---

Beware of "Anti-AIDS" cults

You just got hit with an HIV diagnosis so you're probably seeking answers or comfort. You may be more susceptible to ideas that, under better circumstances, would make little sense. "Antiestablishment" ways of thinking might seem appealing now; they certainly appeal to human nature. People respond to "negative values," such as "don't do this" or "don't do that." Religions and ideologies employ this opposition method to influence behavior. For example, of the Ten Commandments, only two are "positive values." The rest declare "thou shalt not do this" or "thou shalt not do that."

Negative values resonate with people far more than positive values. Political campaigns are always "anti-this" or "anti-that." The makings of an idea—and its opposition—are all around us: anti-Americanism, anti-abortion, or anti-discrimination. A successful "anti-anything" campaign needs a good scapegoat, someone or something to blame the problem on.

One surprisingly popular "anti-AIDS" group is called Health Education AIDS Liaison (HEAL). Once considered an odd fringe group founded in the 1980s, HEAL has grown in numbers and has become relatively influential. The group's mission is to provide "information and support for alternative and holistic approaches to AIDS and related conditions." Chapters are based throughout the United States and Canada, with some local chapters hosting "support" groups.

HEAL has adopted the claims of Duesberg, its battle cry being that people with HIV can stay healthy through "nontoxic, alternative treatments." The group suggests that lifestyle, malnutrition, vaccinations, recreational drugs, illegal street drugs, prescription drugs—including antibiotics and antivirals—sexually transmitted diseases, and psychological and emotional traumas are the true cause of AIDS.

Fringe groups generally rely on scapegoats to fuel their fire. HEAL's pick is the medical establishment and the pharmaceutical industry, which are purportedly in cahoots in a plot to sell "poison" to people for profit. Of course, some lifestyle issues, drugs, and sexually transmitted diseases play a role in good health, but they are not the cause of AIDS. The cause of AIDS is HIV. But if you ask members of HEAL the same question you'll get old research, circular reasoning, and "antiestablishment" philosophies.

Skepticism of established practices can be good. It helps keep some social systems from becoming stagnant. But the danger of cultlike groups like HEAL and other alternative health fanatics, which often prey on the newly diagnosed, is that they twist a few interesting ideas to excess and take advantage of the natural human desire for hope and camaraderie in the face of difficult circumstances.

Having HIV is certainly a difficult circumstance. Learning the news can be incredibly trying. It's natural to have fears and questions about HIV, and it's healthy to have some skepticism about the pharmaceutical industry and the medical community.

However, adopting the philosophies of fanatical groups in place of sound medical advice can have serious and possibly irreparable consequences for your health and well-being. Any extremist group—whether it's on the "alternative" health end of the spectrum or the medical end—should also be viewed with skepticism, especially when the consequences can be detrimental to your health and well being.

IN A SENTENCE:

> *When you hear or learn anything about HIV, consider what's real, what's just an opinion, and what are the true motives of the source.*

living

Alternative Medicine: Vitamins and Supplements

YEARS AGO, I knew this guy who wrote a column for a neighborhood newspaper. After being diagnosed with HIV, he devoted much of his column to hyping alternative medicine as a valid treatment option for HIV. Over the years, I read his column with an open mind. After all, I was in the same boat. I, too, wondered about the role of alternative medicine.

Ultimately, we took different paths when it came to treating HIV. Over the years, I kept up with his column. He often discussed Chinese herbs and even espoused some "cleansing regimen" that was supposed to eliminate toxins. He claimed it boosted his immune system, which then would fight the virus. With time, however, his health declined, as did his faith in alternative medicine. In his last column, he regretted not having pursued conventional HIV treatment sooner.

It's hard to say what role alternative medicine had in his death. In fact, it's hard to say much at all about alternative medicine because there's usually very little science to back up the claims of the people who profit from this industry. What is a fact is that Americans love alternative medicine, scientifically proven or not.

In this country, individuals pay more out of their own pocket for alternative medicine than they do to see a doctor. One study found that almost half of Americans visit an alternative medicine practitioner during a given year. Like it or not, alternative medicine has a role in living with HIV because, well, Americans keep buying and ingesting everything from St. John's Wort to goat serum.

The terms *alternative*, *complementary*, and *unconventional* therapy cover several philosophies and approaches. Some approaches are consistent with Western medicine; some are not. Some therapies are so far outside accepted medical practice that they're difficult to evaluate.

Alternative therapy works in some ways

Does alternative medicine work? It depends on what you mean by *work*. If you mean in a capitalistic way, yes, alternative medicine works quite well. The business of alternative medicine is a booming industry, generating some $27 billion a year (to give you some perspective, consider that the pharmaceutical giant Abbott Laboratory generated just under $18 billion in 2002).

Studies have been conducted on why Americans pursue unproven remedies: The top reasons are relief from chronic conditions that include back problems, anxiety, depression, and headaches. For these specific conditions, alternative medicine probably has a role. However, for directly fighting HIV, nothing has yet stood the test of time.

A few studies on alternative medicine and HIV have been published. One study looked at Chinese herbs to treat HIV. The "treatment" was a combination of about a dozen herbs, all of which had been—and still are—highly touted for boosting the immune system and helping with HIV disease. The study was a large, placebo-controlled clinical trial, conducted in five major cities around the United States. According to Daniel S. Berger, M.D., medical director of Northstar Medical Center in Chicago, the results of the trials demonstrated no reduction in HIV and no immune-related benefits for any of the patients in the trial.

"One should be very careful about not getting dragged into the advertising campaigns made by the companies that produce these products," says Dr. Berger. "One can go into a health food store and the shelves are full of supplements and vitamins which are bandied in front of the customers, touted as 'good for this' and 'good for that.' You're liable to walk out of the health food store with a shopping cart full of medications. You can spend hundreds or thousands of dollars easily." His message: "Beware."

Consider your motivation for alternative medicine

Having HIV is certainly an understandable reason for anxiety or depression or headaches. So it's no surprise that two-thirds of people with HIV use some form of alternative medicine, including yoga, herbal remedies, massage, megavitamins, folk remedies, energy healing, and homeopathy.

But let's be perfectly clear: Alternative therapy does not improve the course of HIV disease. In the last twenty years, numerous attempts have tried to make the connection that alternative medicine improves HIV. By all accounts, they have failed to show a positive connection. And some alternative therapies are dangerous and can make HIV worse.

If you're considering alternative therapies, first consider your motivations. Are you seeking alternative medicine to fight HIV or to make you feel better in a general sense? The distinction is important. For example, if you're secretly harboring hope that Chinese herbs will raise your T-cell count or lower your viral load, you will be disappointed. Hundreds of thousands of people with AIDS have tried this approach throughout the epidemic.

"I had a lot of patients who spent a huge amount of money doing [alternative] things to extremes and still got very sick," says Dr. Berger. He explained that some patients even refused to take conventional HIV treatment and, instead, relied on "high-dose" vitamins and supplements. "They ended up dying," he said.

That was years ago. Today, standard HIV medicine is dramatically improved. There's no good reason—anymore—to look to unproven therapies to keep you healthy. However, if certain forms of alternative medicine—say, yoga, massage, or chiropractic—improve your quality of life and you can afford them, by all means have a field day. Just understand, they don't work for fighting HIV.

For some people, alternative medicine represents a kind of coping strategy, a way to emotionally grapple with a grim situation. "In the old days, when there weren't a lot of [conventional and effective HIV] treatments, patients were desperate, everyone was desperate," says Berger. For combating HIV, Berger said that most of the alternative approaches "don't do much."

Herbal and dietary supplements can be risky

If you like gambling, you'll love herbal medicine. Most herbal or plant-based medicines haven't been properly tested, so they are risky. "Natural" simply means "found in nature." That doesn't mean it's good for you. The poison arsenic is all-natural. If you're taking prescription drugs, be careful about taking herbs or supplements. Some herbs interact with prescription drugs and lead to bad things.

At first, it might make sense that trying to boost your immune system is a way to fight HIV. There's an ongoing war between HIV and the immune system. The immune system can keep HIV in check for many years. But the ongoing battle taxes the immune system.

At some point, the immune system starts to wear down. What it probably needs is a break from the battle and some time to rest and regenerate. It can't rest when HIV is present. The immune systems of some people with HIV eventually burn out.

HIV is a unique virus because it actually feeds on the immune system. When your immune system is activated, HIV is also activated. The virus replicates when T-cells become active. So boosting your immune system is simply giving more food to a hungry virus. It's like fighting a gasoline fire with more gasoline.

Some herbs can hurt

There's no shortage of books, products, and herbal supplements that claim to boost your immune system. For some minor viral infections, alternative therapies might be appropriate in the short term. For HIV, however, boosting your immune system is probably not a good long-term strategy.

"Some of these [alternative] medications can cause allergic reactions," says Dr. Berger. "Also, they can cause diarrhea, which reduces the absorption of [conventional HIV] medications." This, he said, can cause the HIV medications to fail. "So taking herbs or supplements may not be harmless."

If you are taking any medicine—HIV treatment included—you should know about potential interactions between the drugs and herbs. Supplements and herbs are not regulated by the Food and Drug Administration because they are considered food products and nutritional adjuncts, not drugs. As such, the interactions of many alternative products and HIV medicines have not been well studied.

National Center for Complementary and Alternative Medicine

The National Center for Complementary and Alternative Medicine (NCCAM) is a government-sponsored agency for scientific research on complementary and alternative medicine. It's one of the institutes in the National Institutes of Health (NIH). The mission of NCCAM is to explore complementary and alternative healing practices in the context of rigorous science. For more information:

NCCAM, National Institutes of Health

9000 Rockville Pike

Bethesda, Maryland 20892 USA

Web: nccam.nih.gov

Email: info@nccam.nih.gov

Vitamins and botanicals (herbal supplements) to avoid with HIV medicine

St. John's wort

Don't use St. John's wort if you're taking anti-HIV drugs. St. John's wort is a plant product to relieve mild depression. It can cause serious problems when mixed with other medicines including amprenavir, efavirenz, and indinavir. "Patients and health-care professionals need to be aware of this interaction. Most people taking medications to treat HIV infection should avoid using St. John's wort," says AIDS research clinician Judith Falloon, M.D., of the Laboratory of Immunoregulation, National Institute of Allergy and Infectious Diseases (NIAID).

Garlic supplements

"In the presence of garlic supplements, blood concentrations of saquinavir decreased by about 50 percent among our study participants," says NIAID's Falloon. "We saw a definite, prolonged interaction. The clear implication is that doctors and patients should be cautious about using garlic supplements during HIV therapy."

Grapefruit or grapefruit juice

Grapefruit juice is one of the foods most likely to cause problems with drugs because the fruit juice is *hepatically metabolized* and it interferes with more than fifty medications, including HIV medicine.

High-dose vitamin C

High doses of vitamin C reduce the levels of some HIV medicines, specifically a protease inhibitor called indinavir.

Echinacea, ginseng, and ginkgo biloba

Researchers at the National Institutes of Health are assessing potential side effects of echinacea, ginseng, or ginkgo biloba when taken with lopinavir and ritonavir. Until the study is completed, avoid these botanicals when taking HIV medicine.

Milk thistle

Although some studies conducted outside the United States support claims of oral milk thistle to improve liver function, there is no conclusive evidence to prove its claimed uses to this day. The National Center for Complementary and Alternative Medicine (NCCAM) is planning further studies of milk thistle for chronic hepatitis C and HIV patients.

Consult an HIV-experienced professional before taking herbs or supplements

How do you make reasonable decisions about herbs and supplements? Daniel S. Berger, M.D., notes that there are few options. "If your physician happens to be savvy, or somewhat knowledgeable regarding supplements, vitamins, and minerals, you should definitely consult with your physician. If your physician isn't, then consult with a nutritionist that's HIV-knowledgeable."

Berger cautions people not to pursue the herbal or supplement route on their own. "A lot of articles and information on the Internet are done by publicists or people who are trying to increase revenue for companies that are selling the products." Just because information is on the Internet doesn't make it valid.

Put aside the question of the effectiveness of alternative medicine. A more important question is: How are you going to pay for it? Except for chiropractic and sometimes acupuncture, chances are good that it's not covered by health insurance. If committing to a course of some herb or supplement, don't forget you'll be paying for it over the long haul. Small expenses begin to add up when $35 a month becomes $420 a year.

Alternative medicine helps the mind

If you're looking for ways to reduce stress, anxiety, or depression—and the symptoms that stem from these underlying conditions—chances are much better you'll find some alternative medicines beneficial.

YOGA

Yoga is a general term for several spiritual practices that are designed to help people achieve a "higher consciousness" and liberation from suffering. The basic concept behind yoga is that one can gain a better perspective by practicing certain behaviors. Hatha is the most popular type of yoga in the United States and it emphasizes physical control and postures. Yoga has been shown to help with depression, anxiety, heart disease, high blood pressure, headaches, and some forms of chronic pain. It has not been shown to have a direct impact on HIV.

It's hard to explain the benefits of yoga. Some people say it reduces stress by stretching tense muscles and relaxing tight spines. Other people suggest that the mental concentration required by yoga allows them to forget about the worries of daily life. Most people just say they feel better after doing yoga.

A good place to start yoga is in a group class. Most AIDS services organizations can direct you to a reputable yoga class or instructor. Often, such classes are free to people with HIV. If you're new to yoga, take a beginner's class. You'll be surprised how physically demanding it can be.

MASSAGE

Who doesn't feel better after a good massage? There's some evidence that speaks to the reparative qualities of massage. But if you've ever had a good, or at least an enthusiastic massage, then you shouldn't need to be convinced about the merits of massage. At its simplest, massage gives the feeling of general relaxation, as tight muscles are pulled and stretched. Massage styles can range from gentle rocking to intense deep-tissue kneading.

There's an aspect to massage that extends beyond simple pushing and pulling of muscles. Some people say the value-added benefit to massage therapy is the human element. They say some of the potency of massage comes from the instinctual desire to touch and be touched. Babies die without the coddling of an adult. So it makes intuitive sense that expressions of affection such as touching, rubbing, holding, and squeezing are good, not just for the body, but for the soul.

CHIROPRACTIC

Chiropractic medicine attempts to restore normal function of the body by manipulation and treatment of the body structures, especially the back. Through manipulation, chiropractors may be able to relieve joint stiffness and pain. Studies have unequivocally shown chiropractic to be effective for acute lower back pain.

MEDITATION

Meditation uses deep breathing or other techniques to tune out the day-to-day mental chatter and thereby lower anxiety and stress. Some research has shown that meditation can bring about a lowering of heart rate, a decrease in respiration, a decrease in levels of a stress hormone called cortisol, and an increase in brain waves associated with relaxation. Some physicians, therapists, and healthcare workers recommend meditation as a way to relax.

ACUPUNCTURE

This therapy involves the painless insertion of thin needles into the skin to balance the body's flow of energy, referred to as **qi** ("chee"). Acupuncture is sometimes used to relieve neuropathy, fatigue, anxiety, and pain. Acupuncture has been studied for a specific type of pain called HIV-related peripheral neuropathy. It was shown to be no more effective than placebo.

IN A SENTENCE:

> *Herbs and supplements do not work for treating HIV, but some forms of alternative medicine help with symptoms of anxiety and depression.*

learning

Understanding T-Cell Counts and Viral Load Tests

THERE ARE two kinds of blood tests worth paying attention to:

- ○ HIV viral load
- ○ CD4+ cell count (T-cell count)

Consider these tests, also known as **surrogate markers,** as important as a compass and the North Star were to ancient sailors. The results of these two tests will greatly influence your treatment options.

The viral load test measures *how fast* HIV disease is progressing, and the T-cell count reflects *how far* HIV disease has progressed. In general, it's a good thing when your T-cell count is high and your viral load is low or undetectable. On the other hand, it's a bad thing when your T-cell counts are low or your viral load is high.

Imagine a car. Think of your T-cells as the gasoline in the car. The faster you drive, the faster you run out of gas. However, if you start out with a full tank of gas, driving for a long time is no problem. In the same way, if your T-cells are high, living a long time is a given.

Using this example, your viral load is like the speed of the car. The higher the viral load, the faster the disease is progressing. If your viral load is high, it's like you're speeding—and when you run out of gas will depend on what's in your tank. If you're speeding and your T-cells are higher, you've got a ways to go. If you're speeding and your T-cells are low, you're asking for trouble.

	High	Low
T-cells:	good	bad
Viral Load:	bad	good

T-cells are a barometer of your immune system

T-cells are special cells found in your blood. They make up the biggest part of your immune system. Without T-cells, your immune system couldn't fight the viruses, bacteria, and fungi that constantly invade the body. In a twist of fate, T-cells are the most popular target for HIV. The virus infects the very cell designed to fight it.

In healthy people without HIV, the CD4+ T-cell count is generally somewhere between 500 and 1,200 cells per cubic millimeter of blood. A cubic millimeter is equal to about one drop of blood. This measurement is often shortened to ml or mL. A T-cell count of 450 might be written as CD4 = 450 ml.

In the absence of HIV medicine, the T-cell count decreases an average of about 50 to 100 cells each year. The critical threshold for your T-cells is around 200. At that point, it seems, the body becomes especially vulnerable to infections.

T-CELLS 500 OR ABOVE—HIGH

If your T-cells are in this range, it means that HIV has done minimal damage to your immune system.

T-CELLS 499 TO 200—MID-RANGE

A count in this range means that HIV has already caused a mild to moderate amount of damage to your immune system.

T-CELLS 199 TO 0—LOW

If your count falls in this range, it means that HIV has done severe damage to your immune system. If your count falls in this range, you should be taking special antibiotics to prevent a certain type of pneumonia often referred to simply as **PCP**.

How should you feel about your T-cell count?

There are some important things to know about these T-cell counts. A single T-cell count does not mean as much as several T-cells counts taken over time. For example, it's impossible to tell from a single test if your T-cells are rising or falling. Also, T-cell counts naturally fluctuate somewhat. They can be lower if you have a cold or flu when you take the test or higher if your immune system is activated for some reason. The best indicator of your immune system is the overall trend of your T-cell counts over time.

Still, if your T-cell count is lower than you hoped it would be, you're bound to be disappointed. It's all too easy to fixate on a low T-cell count. The news might even lead you to feel nervous or anxious. At first, you may seem okay when hearing that your T-cells are low. But later, you might feel overwhelmed, you might cry, or even find yourself seeking distractions like drugs or alcohol.

There's no one-size-fits-all way of responding to your first T-cell count. In general, if your T-cells are in the high range, you should feel good that you've caught your HIV earlier, before it had a chance to cause much damage. If your T-cells are in the middle range, don't panic. But pay attention by closely monitoring your counts. If your T-cells are low, you should be concerned and you should be taking medications to prevent certain opportunistic infections.

Whatever your T-cell count, it's still only half the picture. The T-cell count can tell you how much damage has already been done to your immune system. It cannot tell you how quickly the damage is being done. The second part of the equation is the HIV viral load.

Viral load is a snapshot of the virus

Before HIV viral load testing was available, doctors and researchers thought the virus stayed dormant for several years after initial infection. However, researchers used viral load testing to learn that, in fact, the immune system and virus are locked in a fierce battle from day one.

Generally speaking, viral load testing employs a technology that finds and amplifies small particles of **DNA**. HIV doesn't have DNA but rather a similar material called **RNA**. The HIV viral load test finds bits of RNA that come from HIV. The test then amplifies the RNA so that it can be measured. The RNA would be impossible to measure unless it was amplified.

There are two main types of viral load tests available: **PCR** and **bDNA**. The abbreviation PCR stands for polymerase chain reaction, and bDNA stands for branched-chain DNA.

The tests are sometimes used for different stages of HIV disease. PCR is the most sensitive and can detect very low levels of virus in the blood, but the bDNA test has been shown to be the most accurate in measuring high levels of virus. Keep in mind that every test has some level of error.

Viral load seems to be a good predictor of disease progression. Viral load tests use the word "copies" to refer to the unit of measurement. For example, a person may get a viral load result of 60,000 copies. Keep in mind that viral copies are measured exponentially. This is different than your T-cell count, which is measured in a linear way, more like the gasoline gauge on your car. For example, the difference between 60,000 and 6,000 is ten times less or 90 percent less. The difference between 60,000 copies and 60 copies is a hundred times less or 99 percent less.

Sometimes, doctors will refer to **log drops** in viral load. A log drop basically means a 90 percent reduction in the level of virus. So, the difference between 60,000 and 6,000 is a one-log drop. The difference between 60,000 and 600 is a two-log drop. A one-log reduction from 150,000 copies to 15,000 copies is the same thing as, say, a one-log reduction from 50,000 to 5,000 copies. Don't worry if this doesn't make a lot of sense right now.

For viral loads, less is better

A high viral load is bad. It literally means that there's more virus in your blood and that the disease is progressing quickly. A low viral load is considered a good thing. It means there's less virus in your blood and the disease is progressing more slowly. Most sensitive viral load tests can measure down to 50 copies of virus. If there are 49 copies, the result will be "undetectable." Clearly, the virus is not gone, it's just below what the test can detect.

People with viral load levels over 100,000 copies are ten times more likely to get sick over the next five years as compared to those with levels below 100,000 copies. Furthermore, people with constant viral load levels below 10,000 seem to have a much lower risk of disease progression. But it doesn't mean that the disease won't progress, it only means that the chance of its progressing is lower.

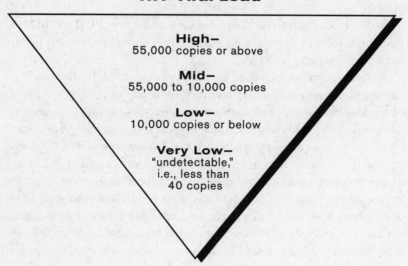

HIV Viral Load

High—
55,000 copies or above

Mid—
55,000 to 10,000 copies

Low—
10,000 copies or below

Very Low—
"undetectable,"
i.e., less than
40 copies

In the normal progression of HIV disease, viral levels tend to rise slowly. As in the case of T-cell counts, a viral load test can vary. Other infections can cause a temporary increase in HIV levels. Some doctors may take two viral load tests, about two to four weeks apart, to establish a baseline level. Tests can vary slightly in their results, so if you're using a particular test you should continue to use the same test.

T-cell plus viral load equals immune strength

Using both T-cell counts and viral load testing gives you and your doctor a more complete picture of your health and the status of your immune system. While T-cell counts reflect your body's firepower for fighting disease, viral load tests indicate the activity of the virus. So what do these tests mean for your life right now? Here's a chart to help you organize your thoughts:

T-cells + Viral Load	Possible Meanings
High + Low	Your immune system is in good shape and the virus seems to be suppressed for some reason. Celebrate, this is great news. Monitor your T-cells and viral load every three to four months.
High + High	Your immune system is still in good shape, but it's not likely to stay that way. Since the virus is active, your immune system is likely to break down soon.
Low + Low	In this case, damage has been done in the past, but the virus is currently being held in check.
Low + High	Not good. Your immune system is damaged and your body is vulnerable to other infections. The virus is replicating quickly, further depleting your immune system.

IN A SENTENCE:

A viral load test measures how fast HIV disease is progressing and a T-cell count reflects how far HIV disease has progressed.

FIRST-MONTH MILESTONE

By the end of the first month, you're beginning to get a handle on how to cope with many issues involved with having HIV:

O YOU KNOW WHY IT'S IMPORTANT TO SHOP AROUND BEFORE CHOOSING AN HIV DOC-TOR, HOW TO MAKE THE MOST OF YOUR LIMITED TIME WITH THAT PERSON, AND HOW HIV AFFECTS THE IMMUNE SYSTEM.

O YOU UNDERSTAND THAT TELLING OTHER PEOPLE ABOUT YOUR HIV STATUS IS ALWAYS YOUR OWN DECISION, ONE THAT SHOULD BE CAREFULLY CONSIDERED BEFOREHAND.

O WHEN YOU HEAR OR LEARN ANYTHING ABOUT HIV, YOU KNOW TO CONSIDER WHAT'S REAL, WHAT'S JUST AN OPINION, AND WHAT'S THE TRUE MOTIVE OF THE SOURCE OF INFORMATION.

O YOU HAVE LEARNED THAT HERBS AND SUP-PLEMENTS DO NOT WORK FOR TREATING HIV, BUT SOME FORMS OF ALTERNATIVE MEDICINE CAN HELP WITH ANXIETY AND DEPRESSION.

○ YOU HAVE BEEN INTRODUCED TO THE MEANING OF A VIRAL LOAD TEST, WHICH MEASURES HOW FAST HIV DISEASE IS PROGRESSING, AND TO THE MEANING OF A T-CELL COUNT, WHICH REFLECTS HOW FAR HIV DISEASE HAS PROGRESSED.

Dating and Sex

DATING ISN'T easy. Even in the best of circumstances, courtship is complicated. Inevitably, the interaction is charged with emotions and expectations. Introduce the wild card of HIV, and the stakes get raised. And for couples in which only one person has HIV, the delicate ritual is even more fragile.

Some relationships between HIV-positives and negatives survive and some don't. Many just never happen to begin with. The pairing of opposites is possible, but it takes work—plenty of work. Now that you know you have HIV, the search for Mr. or Ms. Right may seem impossible. You might have fears of rejection. You might feel like a biohazard or damaged goods.

Many people may choose to shut down or simply take themselves off the market, opting out of dating altogether. These are normal responses, especially early on after an HIV diagnosis. These feelings usually subside with time.

Ultimately, HIV shouldn't deter you from the pursuit of romance. Plenty of HIV-positive people go on to have successful relationships, marriages, and even families. You may not be ready to get involved with another person right away, but it's a relief to know it is possible.

. . .

Issues can emerge for both parties

In the dating world, problems are likely to come up for you and your partner. The fear of contagion is quite real for both partners. For the HIV-negative person, the issue is how to avoid becoming infected. For the positive partner, the fear is of giving the virus to the other person—something that might seem unforgivable. For many HIV-positive people, a little voice inside their head constantly monitors and restricts their every movement.

It's possible to test the dating waters with other HIV-positive people. However, many people are perfectly comfortable dating someone who is HIV-negative. Either way, finding the right time to disclose the news isn't easy. Furthermore, people have very different thoughts on the matter.

Rosetta M., an HIV educator from Buffalo, New York, is the kind of person who discloses her HIV status sooner rather than later. "I wanted to find out who would stand and who would fall away," says Rosetta M. "I realized I didn't need everybody, but I needed a few 'somebodies.' The only way to find them was to let them know who I was. HIV is part of who I am."

Not everyone is as forthcoming. Some people choose to disclose their HIV status after having sex. "I always have safe sex, so it wasn't like I put anyone in danger," says Alan G. "But I told [the person whom I had sex with] over the phone and he freaked. Subsequent phone calls from the guy were threatening. I didn't know what to do. The last time we spoke, I listened to his frustrations and analyzed them. I'm still not sure who to tell on the first date. Sometimes I do, sometimes I don't."

"I couldn't imagine even accepting a date from a person who didn't know I was HIV-positive," says Rosetta. "I let a lot of people know. I knew that when people asked me out, they already knew." In fact, Rosetta is now married to a man who is HIV-negative. "We made eye contact for six months. Then we started to date. Within four months, he realized what an awesome person I was and wanted to marry me."

It always takes two to tango. From the perspective of someone who's HIV-negative, dating a person who is positive may be too scary. There's no shortage of stories about people who were rejected because of their HIV status. But there are also a few success stories.

"My roommate kept telling me about a guy who I would really like, but that I shouldn't go out with him because he suspected that the guy was HIV positive," says Brian K., who is HIV-negative. "Well, I did meet him and we fell in love. He is now my partner. He told me on our second date, before we had a chance to have sex. It didn't hinder my dating him at all. We have been together now for four years. He is a wonderful man."

Steven G. tells a similar story. "My partner worries about getting HIV from me, but ultimately he overlooks it," he says. "I guess he must think I'm worth the sacrifice."

Disclosure Tactics

NOT SURE how to break the HIV news to a date? Here are some personal accounts of how to handle disclosure:

○ I have always told on the first date, sitting across from the person, looking them in their face. Not on the phone, where rejection comes easily. Not in a bar, where alcohol and music can prevent any real conversation. First date, face to face. If he rejects me, he would have had to do so the adult way, the brave way, looking at me, having talked to me and gotten to know me.

○ I don't disclose a thing about HIV until I get to trust the person. I try to get a sense if the person is okay with HIV stuff or not. I drop a hint by saying a good friend of mine has AIDS. I carefully watch how he responds to the hint. You'd be surprised at what you can learn from body language.

○ I make no big secret of my status. It's part of who I am. It's not the only part, so I don't put it in front of my name. But I couldn't imagine a first date going by without this disclosure. At the end of the day, you have to look at yourself in the mirror.

○ I always tell before I'm asked. I indicate my HIV status before I ask others.

Put your emotions aside when thinking about sex

Many people with HIV worry about infecting others. For some people, these worries may even escalate to intense conflict or anxiety. The best way to deal with these concerns is to learn how HIV is transmitted and be honest with yourself about your own sexual behavior.

You might feel awkward or a little guilty when thinking about sex. In fact, you may find yourself wanting to avoid the topic altogether. While reading the remainder of this chapter, put aside your emotions about sex. Emotions don't transmit HIV—specific sexual behaviors do. For now, consider how these behaviors might affect other people. Deal with your emotions about sex later.

A word of caution about discussing sex: Be very selective about the people in whom you confide. Emotions, personal and religious biases, and even outright hostility can surface in people, even in those who may be close to you. Sex and morality are hot-button issues with almost everyone.

People have vastly different opinions about sex and HIV. I've had many acquaintances, some friends, and even professional counselors react negatively or disapprovingly to the idea that HIV-positive people should pursue sex. Make no apologies for wanting a full sex life, just be cautious about the people with whom you discuss the topic.

There will always be isolated stories about someone who apparently got HIV in some obscure way. Don't give in to this sensationalism. The bottom line is that, in terms of sex, the primary way for you to pass HIV is through blood or semen that gets inside another person. This can happen through the anus (a.k.a. the rectum) or vagina. It is very unlikely, but still possible, to pass the virus through genital-to-mouth contact.

The difference between "safe sex" and "safer sex" is just a letter

It's impossible to precisely define "safe" and "unsafe" sexual behavior. In reality, there's only gray area—a continuum of choices—between the two extremes. Among the politically correct crowd, the term *safe sex* is supposed to be a no-no. The correct term to use is *safer sex*. But regular people don't always speak in politically correct terms. So, from here on, I'll refer to *safer* sex as *safe* sex because that's the way we all speak in normal conversations and the difference is only the words, not their meanings. After you understand the realities of how HIV is transmitted, you'll need to weigh the risks and benefits to yourself and to your potential sex partners.

Masturbation is safe sex

Of course, masturbation is the act of stimulating your own genitals using your own hands or other objects, often to the point of orgasm. It's normal and healthy, despite various claims to the contrary. Most everyone masturbates, whether or not they admit to it.

Solo masturbation—without physical contact with another person—is one of the only sexual activities that carries no risk of giving or getting sexually transmitted diseases, including HIV.

The Facts:

HIV LIVES IN:
blood
semen (commonly called cum)
pre-cum (fluid that drips from the penis during arousal)
vaginal fluids
menstrual blood (blood from a woman's period)
breast milk

YOU CANNOT GET HIV THROUGH:
saliva
sweat
urine
feces (as long as blood is not present)
skin-to-skin contact (as long as there are no cuts, abrasions, or sores)

If you have the virus, solo masturbation is a great way of getting sexual pleasure without all the complications that come with another person. In fact, some people masturbate simply to relieve stress or boredom. Whatever the reason, masturbating is completely safe.

Some people carry around subconscious messages from religious backgrounds or from parents that lead to guilt or uncomfortable feelings about masturbating. But don't let that stop you.

For men, using a lubricant during masturbation can help prevent soreness to the penis. There are lots of great "lubes" on the market; look for those that are water-based since they wash off the body easily (and are safe to use with latex condoms). Hand lotion or Vaseline can be used to masturbate, but remember, these contain oils that can damage condoms.

Semen can transmit HIV, so be aware of where your semen ends up. After ejaculation, there will probably be semen on your genitals or your hands. Most guys clean up with a towel, napkin, or even clothing. Both men and women should avoid sharing dildos or sex toys with other people as small amounts of blood, semen, or vaginal secretions might remain on them. If other people use the same dildo or toys as you, it's unlikely but still possible to transmit HIV this way. If you do share toys, wash them well with warm soapy water.

Is getting "head" safe?

Can you pass HIV to another person through oral contact or oral sex? It is possible, but very unlikely. A study published in 2002 found that getting HIV from oral contact with someone's penis is a very rare event. The study looked at men who have sex with men, who exclusively performed oral sex as the person who was "giving head." Twenty-eight percent of the men studied knew their partner had HIV and of those, 35 percent reported getting semen in their mouths. None of the men in the study tested positive for HIV.

On the other hand, another recent study funded by the Centers for Disease Control and Prevention (CDC) found that 7.8 percent of recently infected men who have sex with men were "probably infected through oral sex." One problem with this study, however, was that some of the men who became infected had also engaged in other risky behaviors, so it was hard to identify the real cause. Nearly half of the men who did test HIV-positive reported having oral problems, such as occasional bleeding gums.

If someone engages in oral contact with your penis, or gives you a "blow job," here are some things you can do to reduce the risk to other people:

○ avoid being sucked if you have sores or cuts on your penis
○ avoid being sucked if your partner has bleeding gums, sores, or cuts in his or her mouth
○ avoid ejaculating (cumming) in the other person's mouth

Your mouth and someone's penis

If you suck another person's penis, there is very little chance that HIV can get out of your body. There is wide agreement that "giving head" poses an extremely low risk of passing the virus to another person. In other words, don't worry much about giving the virus to someone if *you* give a blow job. A bigger concern for you is catching additional sexually transmitted diseases (the last part of this section offers more details on condoms).

Someone's mouth and your vagina

Mouth-to-vagina contact is often referred to as "going down," "eating out," or "eating pussy." A less-common term is **cunnilingus**. It's a form of oral sex that involves the stimulation of the vagina by the mouth and tongue, and it's quite common.

If you have HIV and someone's mouth comes into contact with your vagina, the potential risk to that person may come from the discharge of your vaginal secretions, or your menstrual blood, into the mouth of another person.

Studies on the risks of cunnilingus are rare. There are only a few documented cases by the CDC that demonstrate HIV transmission to a person performing oral contact on a woman. This is the best evidence that the risk of transmission through cunnilingus is very low.

It's often suggested that women with HIV use a specially-designed-for-cunnilingus latex barrier called a **dental dam**, or even plastic food wrap (such as Saran Wrap). However, given the potentially low risk of passing HIV by cunnilingus, and the lack of research to document the success of dental dams, most women find them, well, ridiculous.

Someone's mouth and your butt

The act of stimulating the anus by the mouth and tongue is called **anilingus** or more commonly "rimming." The anus has nerve endings in the pelvic region and many people find stimulation to be sexually arousing.

The CDC has clearly stated that fecal matter, in the absence of blood, is not considered to be a bodily fluid that transmits HIV and, therefore, poses minimal risk for transmitting the virus. A potential source of risk for the person who is rimming you would be from very small amounts of blood that may be present in or around your anus. Anal bleeding can occur by prior sexual penetration.

Your mouth and someone's butt

If you "eat" someone's butt (in other words, you do the rimming), there is very little chance that HIV can get out of your body and into theirs. This behavior poses an extremely low risk of passing the virus to another person.

Rimming another person, however, leaves you susceptible to catching additional sexually transmitted diseases. There's considerable risk for contracting hepatitis A and hepatitis B, parasites or "bugs," and a host of other infections.

Urine

Urine does not transmit HIV. Even if the urine contained small amounts of blood, the urine itself would kill the virus.

Your penis and someone's vagina

If you have HIV and you insert your penis in someone's vagina, it's quite possible that you can transmit the virus. In fact, it's the most common way the virus is transmitted in the world. HIV can live in blood, semen, and pre-cum.

The vagina is relatively fragile compared with the mouth. The lining of the vagina can tear and possibly allow HIV to enter a women's body. Tiny cuts or sores inside a vagina can be small or invisible. The virus can pass through the mucous membranes that line the vagina and get inside the woman with whom you're having sex.

For many years, it was believed that an ingredient that was often used in lubricants called **nonoxynol-9** or N-9 might prevent HIV during sexual intercourse. The CDC has declared that N-9 gel does not prevent HIV. In fact, using the N-9 during anal or vaginal intercourse may actually increase the chances that HIV will be transmitted. Some brands of lubricated condoms contain N-9—don't use them.

If you have HIV and you insert your penis into someone's vagina without wearing a latex condom, you are putting that person at a high risk for contracting HIV. Withdrawing your penis before ejaculation is not sufficient protection because of the presence of HIV in pre-cum. The vagina is more susceptible (especially when compared with the mouth), and may allow the virus to get into your partner's bloodstream. You can greatly reduce the risk to your partner by using a latex condom from start to finish (the last part of this section offers more details on condoms).

Someone's penis and your vagina

In general, men are at lower risk of getting HIV from vaginal fluids or menstrual blood. The potential risk comes from vaginal fluid or menstrual blood that comes in contact with the opening of the penis. In fact, some studies have found that, during vaginal intercourse without a condom, a woman with HIV is half as likely to transmit the virus to a man than the other way around. However, the risk increases somewhat if the man has a sore patch of skin on his penis.

If someone comes in contact with your blood during sex, this increases the risk of passing the virus. For example, there may be blood in the vagina if intercourse occurs during a woman's period. You can greatly reduce the risk to your partner by demanding the owner of the penis wear a latex condom from start to finish (the last part of this section offers more details on condoms).

Someone's penis and your butt

There's some controversy about the risks of anal sex or anal-penis contact. If your anus is penetrated by someone's penis—without a condom—the risk of your passing HIV to someone else is minimal, at least when compared with other sexual acts.

The potential risk comes from small, sometimes invisible amounts of blood that come in contact with the opening of the penis or with sore patches of skin on the penis. If someone comes in contact with your blood during sex, this increases the risk of passing the virus. For example, there may be blood in or around your anus if intercourse occurred beforehand. You can greatly reduce the risk to your partner by having that person use a latex condom from start to finish (see the next section of this chapter for details on condoms).

When it comes to anal sex or anal-penis contact without a condom, there is some potential risk to you. This risk comes from the possibility of someone infecting you with a different strain of HIV. In fact, researchers have documented a case of an individual who was infected with a second strain of HIV, one that was more difficult to control.

Your penis and someone's butt

In the continuum between low and high risk, you inserting your penis in someone's anus carries the highest risk for that person. The lining of the anus is even more delicate than the lining of the vagina or the mouth. So it is much more likely to get small cuts or abrasions during sexual contact. Because of this, as well the mucous membranes that line the anus, anal intercourse is a very efficient way to pass the virus.

You can greatly reduce the risk to your partner by using a latex condom from start to finish (see the next section of this chapter for details on condoms). Even if you use a condom, the risk to another person is still relatively higher when compared to oral sex.

Let's be clear, it doesn't matter if you're straight or gay. In fact, researchers have examined the risk for heterosexual HIV transmission to women by HIV-positive men. In couples that engaged in both anal and vaginal intercourse, 62 percent of the cases where HIV transmission occurred were due to anal contact. The researchers reported that the risk for anal contact was 10 times higher than the risk for vaginal contact.

For men who have sex with men, a large study found that about 10 percent got HIV if they engaged in "receptive anal intercourse" (that is, they were the "bottom" partner) with at least two different people over the course of six months. The researchers concluded that "receptive anal intercourse was the only significant risk factor" for getting HIV. This—and many other studies—clearly demonstrate that anal sex without a condom carries the highest risk.

If you have HIV and you insert your penis into someone's anus—without wearing a condom—you are putting your partner at a very high risk for contracting HIV. Withdrawing your penis before ejaculation is not sufficient protection, since pre-cum also contains HIV.

Barebacking happens mostly in the news

There's been a lot of media hype and debate among public health officials about a phenomenon called **barebacking**. The term is defined as intentionally seeking out and engaging in anal intercourse without a condom, whether it's by the "insertive" (top) participant or the "receptive" (bottom) participant. The intentional part distinguishes barebacking from poor planning or spontaneous decisions about not using condoms.

The issue got attention in the gay community, where reports surfaced of a new "subculture" of gay men—mostly HIV-positive—who threw parties, visited sex clubs, and adopted an identity based on the thrill of having sex without condoms. The issue prompted emotional and contentious debates, especially as some speculated that as many as 65 percent of gay men were barebacking.

As it turned out, the issue may have been overblown. In 2002, the CDC announced the results of a large study showing the incidence of barebacking to be only 14 percent. Although the study found that 22 percent of HIV-positive men acknowledged barebacking—versus 10 percent for the HIV-negative group—the majority of HIV-positive men engaged in this activity with other HIV-positive men. Researchers concluded that there is a relatively small number of "hard-core barebackers." Primary motivators included enhanced physical stimulation and emotional connectedness.

An unfortunate fallout from the bareback phenomenon is the public perception of HIV-positive men as irresponsible. As such, health officials have responded with programs and media campaigns that call for men with HIV to always disclose their HIV status to potential sex partners.

At the same time, new studies confirmed that about one in four people in the United States who have HIV are not aware of their own infection. Public health campaigns, however, call for full disclosure of HIV status— an impossible goal if you don't know you have the virus. The most prudent approach for everyone is to practice safe sex as often as possible rather than relying on others to reveal their HIV status. If you have HIV, ultimately what matters is what you do, not what you say.

Using condoms is like wearing seat belts in a car

It would be ideal if everyone used condoms, but, let's be real, not everybody does. If you already have HIV, all the rhetoric you see or hear about wearing condoms to prevent HIV suddenly loses its punch. You've probably been told dozens of times to use condoms for vaginal and anal sex so I won't repeat it.

I will, however, offer you some straightforward reasons on why you should use latex condoms as often as possible:

○ Condoms offer you protection from a long list of nasty STDs— including hepatitis—that can damage your immune system and may shorten your life.

○ Condoms can greatly reduce your chance of getting or giving genital herpes or genital warts (another chapter offers more details on herpes and HPV). While condoms don't entirely prevent the transmission of these diseases, they spin the odds in your favor. There are many strains of both herpes and HPV. Even if you already have one strain, you can still get another.

○ Condoms can prevent you from getting strains of HIV that may be worse than the one you already have. This has been documented (it's called super-infection and you don't want it). You're in this for the long haul, so keeping out unwanted strains of HIV will help you preserve your health in the years to come.

○ Condoms may help you avoid awkward or even illegal situations. You may be too fearful to disclose your HIV status to others—but you can wear a condom without disclosing your status or arousing suspicion in others. Remember, when it comes to sex, what matters most is not what you say, but what you do.

Practice using condoms alone at first

Let's face it, using condoms can be awkward, especially when you're not completely familiar with them. One way to get a "feel" for condoms is to

How to Put on a Condom

STUDIES HAVE shown that condoms break less than 2 percent of the time. Most of the breakage is due to incorrect use, rather than poor condom quality. In case no one has told you how to properly wear a condom, here's a reminder:

1. First off, don't store condoms in a glove compartment or in your wallet; heat and sunlight may damage them. Don't use old condoms or ones that are beyond their expiration date. Don't open them with your teeth and be mindful of fingernails. They can be torn.

2. Most condoms have a small pouch at the tip designed to catch the semen. Put a few drops of water-based lube inside the tip. Force the air from the pouch at the tip of the condom by squeezing it.

3. Put the condom on after the penis is hard. Squeeze the tip of the condom to leave some extra space; but ensure that no air is trapped in the tip. (The water-based lube should fill the space.) Roll the rest down the shaft of the penis. When fully unrolled, the condom should extend almost to the base of the penis.

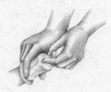

4. If the penis has a foreskin, put the condom on with the foreskin pushed back. Once the shaft is covered, push the foreskin forward (toward the tip). This lets the foreskin move without breaking the condom.

5. Put more water-based lube on the outside of the condom.

6. After ejaculation, the condom should be removed carefully to prevent semen from spilling out. To do this, the penis is withdrawn while holding the condom securely to the penis (so it doesn't get left behind). After removal, dispose of the condom and don't reuse it.

collect several different kinds of them first. Then, try masturbating with them. You'll probably find a specific brand that fits best. Save the package so you remember what brand you'll want to use regularly. Here are some important tips to keep in mind:

- Using oil-based lubricants can weaken latex, causing the condom to break. In addition, condoms can be weakened by exposure to heat or sunlight, or by age. Teeth or fingernails can also tear them.
- Different types and brands of condoms are available from almost any drug store. Remember, only latex condoms stop HIV. Natural membrane ("skin" or "lambskin") condoms are designed to stop pregnancy, not HIV, so don't use them. Female condoms are also available, but their usefulness for HIV has not been well studied.
- Some condoms come with lubrication ("pre-lubed"), others don't. Either way, do not use hand lotion, moisturizer, cold creams, Vaseline, baby oil, mineral oil, vegetable oil, Crisco, or any other products that contain oils. Oils can damage condoms and cause them to break.
- When using condoms, use only water-based lubes. Some water-based lubes include Astroglide, KY, Probe, and Wet. An easy way to tell the difference between oil- and water-based lubes is how they "bead" water. If you're not sure, read the label. If you're still not sure, don't use it.
- For condoms to provide maximum protection, they must be used correctly. Use a new condom each time you engage in sex. Do not use a condom more than once.

IN A SENTENCE:

> *Understand that only certain sexual behaviors can transmit HIV and such behaviors can affect your health and the health of other people.*

learning

Managing Herpes and HPV: New Approaches

Among people with HIV, herpes, and HPV are fairly common. They can be frustrating and distressing, but they also can be treated and managed, or entirely prevented—if you're knowledgeable and open about these topics.

Herpes Simplex Virus—abbreviated as *HSV*—is the blanket name given to a large family of viruses. The herpes family has many different strains, each with its own particular traits. Some strains infect cows, or horses, or monkeys. Some strains of HSV infect only birds (by the way, some people call that condition *chirpies*).

Several varieties of HSV prefer human hosts. For example, *Herpes Simplex Virus Type 1*—abbreviated as *HSV-1*—does a good job at infecting humans, especially around the lips and mouth. In fact, 90 percent of all people have been exposed to HSV-1.

I've had HSV-1 since I was a kid, and it manifests in what people usually call "cold sores." I've been getting cold sores above my upper lip and below my nose since about the age of nine. The outbreaks always start as a tingling sensation and then some pain and tenderness in the area. Within a few hours, a dime-sized cluster of blisters breaks out through the skin.

Although my outbreaks only happen twice a year, I don't like them one bit. They hurt. I feel self-conscious. It's no fun. However, the biggest difference now is that when I feel the familiar tingle, I take an anti-herpes drug right away. The drug makes the outbreaks less severe and the blisters heal faster.

In the past thirty years, an incredible amount of research has been done on herpes. Since 2000, even more research has been done on the interaction between the herpes family of viruses and HIV (which is a member of its own viral family). What researchers and doctors now know is that HIV generally makes HSV worse. But HSV doesn't necessarily make HIV worse.

If you have HSV and you're newly diagnosed with HIV, understand that HSV could become more aggressive, with more severe or more frequent outbreaks. On the other hand, if you have HIV—but don't have HSV—it's wise to keep things that way. Either way, the good news is that HSV (with or without HIV) can be successfully managed by safe and effective drugs.

Genital herpes is extremely common

Genital herpes is yet another name for another member of the herpes family. The generic name of genital herpes is *Herpes Simplex Virus Type 2,* abbreviated as HSV-2. About 30 percent of people in general have been exposed to HSV-2. Among people with HIV, between 50 to 95 percent have been exposed to HSV-2.

Herpes is the most common sexually transmitted disease among people with HIV. According to Daniel S. Berger, M.D., medical director of North-star Medical Center, he sees HSV almost every day during his busy HIV practice in Chicago. "There's not a single day that we don't see herpes infections," says Berger, "and there's not a single week that we don't get a call from a patient with an outbreak."

While HSV-1 is generally milder and tends to affect the mouth and lips, it can certainly occur on or around the genital area. HSV-2 is usually more aggressive and tends to infect the skin on or around the genitals, but it can also infect the mouth and lips. In fact, more and more over the years, the distinction between the two types of herpes is blurring. Both types of herpes are basically treated in the same way: with anti-herpes medication.

One big difference is how society reacts. At a party, admit to someone that you get "cold sores" on your lips and the response will probably be understanding. But admit that you have genital herpes and you'll find people get uncomfortable. Now, throw in the HIV zinger, and you'll probably find yourself standing alone, chewing on a straw. Statistically, however, you're hardly alone.

Symptoms of herpes are not always obvious

For clarity, I'm going to refer to both HSV-1 and HSV-2 collectively as simply HSV. They are transmitted in the same way. They can infect the same parts of the body. And they are treated with same medicine.

With this in mind, about two-thirds of people who have HSV don't know they have the virus. This is either because they have no symptoms or because their symptoms are so mild they go unnoticed. Many people mistake HSV for yeast infections, jock itch, abrasions, insect bites, hemorrhoids, or other skin conditions.

Symptoms of the first HSV infection usually appear one to twenty-six days after being exposed to the virus. At first, some people report flulike symptoms such as swollen glands and fever. This is usually followed by swelling, small sores, or blisterlike lesions on the affected skin. The outbreaks can last a few days or a few weeks. Eventually, the blisters or lesions crust over and new skin tissue forms over them.

Although the blisters on your skin may appear to go away, HSV continues to live in the nerves that supply your skin with feeling. During initial infection on the skin, HSV travels down the nerves, where it hides in a resting state. Then, for a number of reasons, HSV is triggered. It grows back up the nerves and out into the skin, which causes the blisters.

After the initial outbreak, signs and symptoms of herpes can vary greatly from one episode to the next, and from one person to the next. In males, HSV is common on the penis or around the opening of the penis called the urethra. In females, HSV is common around the vagina. Both men and women can get HSV near the anus, on the thighs, buttocks, or anywhere near the genital area. And don't forget that HSV can also infect the lips, mouth, and eyes.

Skin-to-skin contact is how herpes spreads

Both types of HSV are spread by genital-to-genital contact, by mouth-to-genital contact, or by mouth-to-mouth contact.

Herpes can be spread through:

- sexual intercourse (vaginal and anal)
- mouth-to-mouth sexual contact (kissing)

○   close oral, anal, or genital contact
○   mutual masturbation
○   genital-to-genital contact

A person is considered contagious when they have symptoms (the itching and tingling that come before the outbreak of a herpes sore), active sores, and sores that have begun to heal. Herpes can also be spread by the fingers. If enough active virus touches the skin where it is thin (on the mouth, genitals, or eye areas), or where the skin is broken, cut, or scratched, the virus can enter the body. For example, if you have a cold sore and you kiss someone, you can transfer the virus from your mouth to theirs. And if you have a cold sore and put your mouth on another person's genitals, you can infect that person.

Don't forget that herpes can spread from one part of your body to another (called *auto-inoculation*) if you touch a herpes sore and then touch another area that will let the virus enter. Herpes only spreads (from one person to another or from one part of your body to another) when the virus is active, not when it's in a resting state.

Drugs to fight herpes are safe and effective

In his HIV clinic, Berger educates his patients to recognize the early warning signs of an HSV outbreak. If you recognize the symptoms early enough, you can take an anti-herpes drug, which eases the outbreak or prevents it entirely.

The three most-used anti-herpes drugs are:

ACYCLOVIR (ALSO CALLED ZOVIRAX)

The generic drug called acyclovir (pronounced "ay-sike-lo-vir") is used to treat HSV. The drug is well studied in people with HIV and without. Like other antiviral drugs, acyclovir does not rid the body of HSV, but reduces the ability of the virus to grow. As anti-herpes drugs go, acyclovir has a very good record as being safe and effectiveness. According to Berger, if the outbreak is not complicated and someone has easier access to the generic brand—as opposed to the brand name Zovirax—then generic acyclovir is ideal. Acyclovir tablets often come in 800 mg strength, taken up to five times a day.

Valacyclovir (also called Valtrex)

Valacyclovir (pronounced "val-a-sike-lo-vir") is a fancy and more expensive version of acyclovir. But it has been studied and proven effective in suppressing genital herpes outbreaks among people with HIV. One study showed that after six months, the proportion of patients who did not have an outbreak was 80 percent in those taking the drug, compared to only 38 percent of those receiving placebo. Another study showed that the drug lengthened the time between recurrences—for both oral and genital herpes.

Famciclovir (also called Famvir)

A similar drug for HSV is called famciclovir (pronounced "fam-sike-lo-vir"), of which its brand name is Famvir. This drug has been studied in people with HIV. "Famvir has the best tissue penetration of all three of the herpes medicines," says Berger. Studies have shown that taking Famvir very early in the outbreak of HSV (within six hours), you can dramatically slow or stop the virus to prevent a full outbreak. Famvir is usually prescribed as two 500-mg tablets taken as soon as you feel the outbreak, and then take another two 500-mg tablets about twelve hours later.

Topical creams

Topical creams for HSV contain very small amounts of anti-HSV drugs mixed into a benign cream. According to Berger, if somebody has a small outbreak on their lip, you can use topical cream. A friend of mine swears by an over-the-counter cream called Abreva. However, buying a topical cream is expensive, so Berger suggests a cheaper and more effective alternative: Take an anti-herpes pill and crush it up in a bowl, add one or two drops of water, make a paste from the mixture. Then just smear it right on the blisters. "It's much more effective and doesn't cost anything."

"Herpes is very easily treated," says Berger. "The medication that's used for herpes is very benign, with few side effects." If you think you're getting an outbreak, Berger advises not to wait for the blisters to appear before taking anti-herpes medicine.

For many people, outbreaks can be so emotionally distressing or so severe, it makes more sense to prevent them outright. All the anti-herpes drugs—acyclovir, valacyclovir, and famciclovir—can be taken every day, even when symptoms aren't present. This strategy is called **prophylaxis**, where you take anti-herpes drugs everyday to prevent outbreaks entirely. Unfortunately, herpes prophylaxis doesn't guarantee you'll never get an outbreak. But it can dramatically reduce your chances of getting an outbreak.

Genital warts are caused by a family of viruses called HPV

One of the biggest success stories in medical history is directly due to George Papanicolaou. He was a cancer researcher in the early 1900s. He discovered that cancer of the uterus could be detected very early, before it spread and got worse. Later in his career, he invented a test—Papanicolaou's test—now known as the *Pap smear*. Because of this test—from 1947 to 1982—the rates of cervical cancer among U.S. women declined by 75 percent. And the death rate from cervical cancer declined by 80 percent.

The Pap smear allows doctors to detect unusual cells growing in the cervix. Sometimes unusual cells are those that are pre-cancerous. One main cause of these pre-cancerous cells is a family of viruses with the generic name of name *human papilloma virus,* or *HPV* for short.

HPV and HSV are similar in that both are spread by skin-to-skin contact. But unlike HSV, which hides in your nerves, HPV stays in the skin, especially warm and moist skin. And instead of producing blisters or lesions, HPV produces cauliflower-like bumps and abnormal growths in the skin. These abnormal growths are exactly what Papanicolaou's test can detect.

There are about a hundred different members of the HPV family. Some strains are worse than others. One type of HPV causes warts on the hands (called palmar warts) and another type causes warts on the feet (called plantar warts). Several types of HPV prefer the warmer, wetter skin of the genitals, hence the name *genital warts*.

All types of HPV can be classified as either cancer-causing or non-cancer causing. One cancer-causing type is HPV-16, which is responsible for about half of all cervical cancers worldwide. HPV-18 causes another 20 percent. The entire family of HPV accounts for 99 percent of all cervical cancers.

In general, the pace at which cancer develops in the cervix is slow. Once HPV infects the area around the cervix, it lingers in the skin. There, HPV causes molecular changes in skin cells. Over five to 20 years, these changed skin cells become more pronounced, mutating from normal, to pre-cancerous, to cancerous. In people with HIV, the progression tends to happen faster.

Women with HIV should get a Pap smear

How HPV interacts with HIV is the research focus of Joel M. Palefsky, M.D. He's a professor of medicine at the University of California at San Francisco and a renowned clinical expert on HPV-related cervical and anal cancer in people with HIV.

"It's been shown over a number of years and in a number of studies that HIV-positive women are at increased risk of cervical HPV infection," says Palefsky. If you look at HIV-positive women with HPV, and you compare them to similar HIV-negative women, the HIV-positive women are more prone to cervical cancer.

As T-cells decline in HIV-positive women, the risk for cervical cancer increases. One study of women with more than 500 T-cells found about 35 percent had pre-cancerous cells. For women with less than 200 T-cells, more than half had pre-cancerous cells.

The next obvious question for women with HIV: Now what? Over the years, doctors have developed clear guidelines to assess HPV-related cancer risk in women with HIV. These guideline include:

- First get a Pap smear. In fact, all doctors are required to give women with HIV a cervical Pap smear test as part of a first visit. If the results are normal, have the test repeated in six months. If the results are abnormal, don't panic. This can be caused by other conditions. Still, the next step is a visual inspection of the cervix by a physician. This inspection is called a colposcopy, which is a relatively simple and painless procedure, usually performed in the physician's office. Results of the colposcopy will determine your next step.

- Repeat the Pap smear in six months. If the results of both the first and second test are normal, it's okay to continue getting a Pap smear only once a year. If the second test is abnormal, your physician may perform a colposcopy and the results will determine your next step.

- If both the first and second tests are abnormal, and a colposcopy shows potential problems, your physician should begin treatment for HPV itself, or remove the problem-causing cells. Treatment options are discussed later in this chapter.

Pap smears can predict trouble—for women and men

New research in just the last few years is showing that HPV-related cancer in the cervix is very similar to HPV-related cancer in the anus. According to Palefsky, the skin cells in the cervix are biologically similar to the skin cells in the anus. But don't confuse the anus with the rectum. From bottom to top, the anus is the opening part at the lowest end. The rectum is located further up, past the anus. The rectum connects the anus (at the bottom) to the large intestine (at the top). Typical rectal cancer is not related to HPV.

People with HIV have twice the risk of anal cancer when compared to similar people without HIV. If you break this down between HIV-positive men and HIV-positive women, the risk of anal cancer is seven times higher for women and thirty-seven times higher for men. According to Palefsky, the increased risk for both genders is directly related to HPV infection of the anus.

"Virtually everyone who's HIV-positive has anal HPV infection," says Palefsky, "usually with multiple HPV types, typically with at least one [cancer-causing] type." Just as in cervical cancer, when T-cells decline the risk for anal cancer increases. One study found that for men with less than 200 T-cells, almost 75 percent have pre-cancerous cells in the anus. For women, the risk for HPV-related anal cancer was even higher than their risk for cervical cancer. While HPV is typically found in the anus of HIV-positive men, it can be found in both the cervix *and* the anus in HIV-positive women.

Because the skin cells of the anus and the cervix are similar, the model for anal cancer screening is based on the model for cervical cancer screening. This means that to detect cancer in the anus, HIV physicians should perform a Pap smear on the anus. This is a new way of using Papanicolaou's test, so many doctors may not be familiar with this procedure, but more and more this is being accepted as an important screening test for anal cancer.

Being aggressive about HPV-related treatment can pay off

There are no treatments specifically for HPV once you have it, wherever you may have it. However, there are successful treatments to remove the pre-cancerous cells that are caused by HPV. Visible warts should be removed—and sooner is always better. Untreated, the warts are very likely to grow in size or multiply in number. It's possible they may go away on their own, but it's unlikely if you have HIV. Still, research suggests that removing visible warts reduces your chance of getting pre-cancerous or cancerous cells, but it does not eliminate the chance of you spreading HPV to someone else.

There are many ways to treat genital warts and there is no definite evidence to say that any one method is superior. Keeping your T-cells as high as possible, quitting smoking (research has validated this), and finding a health-care professional with experience in treating HPV are probably your best bets. Warts often come back after treatment, so you'll need to be committed to having them treated several times. Don't be discouraged if they come back.

Treatment for genital warts may include one—or a combination—of the following:

- ○ **Podofilox solution or gel**—Podofilox is an corrosive liquid that destroys the problem cells. It should be used on the outside of the anus only.
- ○ **Imiquimod cream (also called Aldara)**—Aldara cream enhances your own body's immune response, which destroys the problem cells. Can cause irritation.
- ○ **Cryotherapy**—This uses liquid nitrogen to freeze and kill the problem cells.
- ○ **Infrared coagulation**—A relatively new treatment that destroys problem cells with a burst of infrared light.
- ○ **Podophyllin**—This treatment is a corrosive lotion or gel that destroys the problem cells.
- ○ **Trichloroacetic acid**—This is an acid that destroys problem cells.
- ○ **Surgical removal**—Basically, a surgeon cuts out the problem cells with a knife. It can be painful and recovery is long.
- ○ **Laser surgery**—A laser is used to destroy the problem cells.
- ○ **Alpha Interferon**—This injection, by needle, enhances your own body's immune response, which destroys the problem cells.

New vaccines can prevent HPV

There is a bright spot to all of this; progress is being made. There are two new—and competing—vaccines to prevent the worst types of HPV. While they don't cure the HPV if you already have it, they are preventive, so if you don't have HPV, you can keep things that way. Both vaccines have been shown to be safe and effective in preventing some types of HPV. The two vaccines are:

GARDASIL IS DESIGNED TO PREVENT HPV TYPES 6, 11, 16, 18

Gardasil, made by Merck, is currently recommended for girls and women between the ages of nine and twenty-six. But new research has started among women older than twenty-six. Time will tell.

CERVARIX IS DESIGNED TO PREVENT HPV TYPES 16 AND 18

Cervarix is intended for women between the ages of fifteen to twenty-five, but the vaccine maker, GlaxoSmithKline has suggested it may work on older women as well.

"But we are not quite out of the woods yet," says Palefsky. "Even if these vaccines are perfect, the best that we can expect is that they'll reduce cervical cancer by about 70 percent." That's important, because women will still need to be screened with Pap smears and followed by a doctor over time because 30 percent will still be at risk.

IN A SENTENCE:

> *Herpes and HPV are common sexually transmitted diseases and there are effective treatments for both.*

living

Anxiety, Depression, and Suicidal Thoughts Are Normal

I TESTED positive for HIV in 1987. During the three months since I had gotten my results, I walked out on my job, quit summer school, and spent most of my time drinking and crying.

The initial shock had subsided, but another emotion began to take its place. At the time, I didn't know there was a specific medical name for what I was feeling. I thought I was just nervous, very nervous. The feeling descended on me when I thought about what was happening. I started sweating, my heart began to race, and I couldn't seem to breathe.

A few belts of gin made the feeling go away. But after three months, I was running out of money and excuses for avoiding my family. The pressure mounted until I couldn't take it any longer. So one evening, I set out for a local AIDS organization that was holding a public meeting.

At the meeting, I didn't talk to a soul. I sat in the back, afraid, and somehow expected other people to approach me. When they didn't, when I left the meeting room, I felt so scared and alone that I wanted to die. Then it occurred to me: Instead of dealing with money, family, and an ugly disease, I would just kill myself.

At a drugstore, I bought some over-the-counter pills and more gin. Back at my apartment, I sat in the dark wondering. Swallowing all those pills was the easy part. The problem was how I felt after they were down. I got really scared in a pathetic kind of way. I curled up on the floor. At least things would be different, if nothing else.

It wasn't until my stomach started convulsing that I completely chickened out and called a friend. He arrived and when we got to the hospital, I was covered in vomit and couldn't stand upright.

In the emergency room, someone shined a light in one of my eyes. I heard something about a stomach pump, and I was restrained in a chair. A tube went down my throat. On first try, it must have gone down wrong, and I started bleeding. On second try, after gagging and gasping for air, the tube went down.

Suicide is not like it is in the movies, where someone takes some pills, has a few drinks, and neatly drifts off to sleep. In reality, it is a messy, painful, degrading, and ultimately an expensive way to get attention. While strapped to that chair, what I remember most was that I didn't want to die at all. I just wanted somebody to help me.

Having HIV is easier these days

Back in 1987, having HIV was a different thing. People were hysterical, there were no treatments, and it really was considered a death sentence. For people testing positive today, everything about the disease is so drastically improved that, by all measures, it's truly a chronic, manageable condition. I am proof of that.

However, breakthroughs in medicine and improved social acceptance of the disease don't always change how people feel when they first test positive. Emotions don't always respond to statistics.

You may be facing any number of challenges in your life beyond HIV. Testing positive might feel like the straw that breaks the camel's back. You may feel a loss of control over your life, or a variety of overwhelming fears. These feelings may hit you all at once, or they may come and go, depending on other factors in your life.

On the other hand, you may be coping well. Perhaps you had expected the diagnosis and were aware of the advances in treatment. Maybe you have friends with HIV who are well and happy. If this is the case, you're lucky. However, don't dismiss the subtle emotional impact that HIV can have as you go about your business.

Either way, understanding your feelings—and knowing how you might respond to certain situations down the road—can help in adjusting better and more quickly to the changes in your life during the next year.

Anxiety, depression, and thoughts of suicide are normal for anyone facing a major medical condition, including HIV. The Living section of this chapter explores some of the typical reactions that people might have after testing positive. The Learning section offers some potential actions and treatments for these conditions.

Above all, if you begin to feel overwhelmed by any emotion, or find yourself in a numb or emotionless state, the most important thing you can do is to ask for help.

Anxiety starts with persistent worrying

Anxiety is not easy to define. It is a disturbance of your mood or emotional tone. It can start as a sense of worry, stress, or nervousness about an anticipated event or outcome.

The likelihood of developing anxiety probably involves life experiences, your psychological makeup, and genetic factors. Men tend to experience more anxiety than women; however, it is not entirely clear why.

Mild-to-moderate anxiety is very common. Symptoms may include excessive worrying, agitation, shakiness, irritability, feeling "on edge" or "hyper," muscle tension, difficulty concentrating or falling asleep, and changes in appetite. Certainly, testing positive for HIV is a major life event and mild-to-moderate anxiety can be expected with varying degrees and at different times.

More pronounced or persistent anxiety can be classified as a medical condition called an anxiety disorder. The lifetime prevalence of anxiety disorders in the United States is between 10 and 15 percent. Reports have confirmed that increased anxiety—often lasting up to several months—are common in the course of living with HIV. However, specific anxiety disorders appear to be no more common in people with HIV than in the general population. Some anxiety disorders include:

○ **Generalized anxiety disorder.** Medically speaking, generalized anxiety disorder is when you persistently have vague feelings that something bad is going to happen. Excessive or unrealistic worries are often so persistent that you cannot make them go away, or you have difficulty concentrating on daily tasks.

○ **Panic disorder.** Panic disorder is when you feel unexpected and repeated episodes of intense fear accompanied by physical symptoms such as your heart beginning to race, chest pains, shortness of breath, dizziness, nausea, numbness, trembling, abdominal distress, and a fear of going crazy or dying. The attack usually hits abruptly, building in intensity within ten to fifteen minutes. You may want to flee from the location where the "panic attack" started. Attacks usually last no more than thirty minutes.

○ **Post-traumatic stress disorder.** Post-traumatic stress disorder usually happens after a terrifying event, causing repeated frightening thoughts and memories. Ordinary events can trigger flashbacks or intrusive images. People may become easily irritated or have violent outbursts. One recent study of ethnically diverse women found up to 42 percent of women who sought treatment for HIV met the criteria for this disorder.

It's normal to worry when you have HIV

If you just found out you have HIV, who could blame you for being worried? But you're not alone in your concerns. The psychological impact of HIV has been well studied by researchers and mental health professionals who have found many common themes. Among them are:

○ **Fear of the unknown.** If you don't know much about HIV, you might believe you won't live much longer.

○ **The unpredictable nature of HIV**. When your blood tests are good, you may feel elated, but when they're down, you may feel worry and anxiety.

○ **Fear of stigmatization.** Gay men, African Americans, and intravenous drug users, and sex-trade workers are already stigmatized by society. You might feel HIV will bring about more labeling, rejection, isolation, or discrimination.

○ **Being a hypochondriac.** You might become obsessed with minor illnesses or fluctuations in your body. You might spend too much time checking your lymph nodes, your skin, or your mouth.

○ **Pressure to maintain a positive attitude.** You might feel as if you should be optimistic all the time. The pressure might be aggravated thinking that self-affirmation, laughter, and positive thinking can control the disease.

Depression can slowly creep into your life

I wish I could report that things got better after my suicide attempt, that I got the help I actually needed, and that it was smooth sailing afterward. But it's rare when big problems in life get fixed in simple ways.

A few months passed. I managed to hold down a job, which helped with finances and kept my mind occupied. I drank less, probably because I conned different doctors into prescribing me tranquilizers. With each doctor, I recited the same sob story about "fear of dying with AIDS." Hence, I maintained a steady supply of sedatives and sleeping pills.

I thought I was coping fairly well with anxiety. However, what seemed to take its place was, well, a lack of emotions, a numbness and apathy. This lack of concern was not just about my health situation, but about life in general. On a good day, my moods were neutral. Slowly and subtly over time, I lost the desire to have fun. Fun was lowering the shades, downing a few tranquilizers, eating Haägen-Dazs, and watching reruns of *I Love Lucy*.

I slept a lot. In fact, I disliked waking. Whenever I woke up, I had a few good moments until I was hit with the reality of my situation. My running joke was that sleeping was the only way to be alive and unconscious at the same time. Soon, I gained weight, felt worse, and the vicious cycle was in motion.

Depression is not sadness, and it is not a character flaw

Depression is more than feeling sad, although people often use the term *depression* to describe sadness. Sadness or the "blues" are actually short-lived, unhappy feelings that occur in response to a particular event. They generally fade with time, or as the event resolves or improves.

As with anxiety, true depression is a chronic medical condition. It's a potentially severe brain-chemical imbalance that interferes with normal functioning—and 15 percent of the time, it resolves by suicide.

Unlike anxiety, depression is about twice as common in women as in men. About one in ten Americans experiences chronic depression, while the rates for people with HIV are estimated at about one in three, making it the most common psychiatric disorder among this group. While just the thought of having HIV may seem depressing, the true underlying reason may be that depression-prone people are more likely to get HIV in the first

Are you depressed?

DOCTORS USE specific guidelines to determine if someone is clinically depressed. If you have five of the following nine symptoms every day for at least two weeks, you're likely to have major depression. You should discuss these symptoms with your health-care provider.

1.   Depressed mood

This isn't just rainy days or Mondays. This is deep, unrelenting sadness that may even "color" the way you see normal things in your life.

2.   Diminished interest or pleasures

When I was depressed, I didn't return phone calls, I didn't make plans with other people, I didn't exercise, and I really didn't care.

3.   Weight changes

Most people lose weight, I gained weight.

4.   Sleeping too much or too little

Persistent changes in your normal sleep patterns may signal depression. If I start sleeping more than my normal eight hours, I know something is wrong.

5.   Restlessness or inactivity

After waking, I would lie around in my robe for hours, smoking cigarettes, drinking coffee, and never got much accomplished. Then, I was late to work.

6.   Fatigue or loss of energy

This is a constant heaviness, particularly in the arms and legs. Some people feel as if they're carrying around a cinder block. I dreaded the idea of climbing stairs, especially with groceries.

7.   Feelings of worthlessness or guilt

Classic symptoms, these feelings may become exaggerated far beyond what people without depression would feel in the same circumstances. I often obsessed about the idea of disappointing my parents.

8.   Inability to think clearly

Most people are a little slow or groggy when they first wake up from sleep. Depressed people may feel as they can't shake off this grogginess all day long.

9.   Suicidal thoughts

Testing positive for HIV makes people think about mortality. Dying or funeral fantasies are human and normal. But when these thoughts persist over time or grow in seriousness, that's not normal.

place. Some research even suggests that HIV itself may play a role in clinical depression. Without question, depression manifests in other chronic viral conditions such as hepatitis B or hepatitis C.

An interesting study recently found that, although death rates among women with HIV have decreased in the United States since the introduction of new HIV treatments, the proportion of deaths caused by non-AIDS-related conditions has remained steady at about 20 percent. Researchers reported that the majority of non-AIDS-related deaths were related to depression and substance abuse.

Depression is not a character flaw. It's not laziness or a lack of motivation. It's an abnormally low level of a brain chemical called **serotonin**, the brain chemical that helps humans cope with stresses from the outside world. Low levels of serotonin are linked to all kinds of unhealthy behavior, such as overeating, aggression, alcoholism, drug addiction, and compulsive behaviors.

If you have five of the symptoms of depression, you're clinically depressed. The next section will discuss some options for you. However, if you have four of these symptoms, that doesn't mean you're fine. Depression can wax and wane, come and go. It's a good idea to write down any symptoms in your health journal and track them over time. This way, you can track any symptoms of depression over time and then discuss them in detail with your doctor. In fact, tracking the details of depression with a health journal may even help you and your doctor decide your next steps.

Many people don't acknowledge depression

Many people see depression as a sign of weakness, so they don't acknowledge the depth of their condition. That's one way to deal with the situation. But research shows that depression is associated with higher rates of mortality in people with HIV. The cause and effect of an HIV diagnosis and depression is not always clear. What's clear is that relief is out there—if relief's what you want. The next section of this chapter is devoted to ways to deal with depression as well as anxiety.

Thinking about suicide is normal, planning it is not

Researchers in France recently discovered that among HIV-positive people who had a good response from HIV treatment, one in ten committed suicide. These were people with high T-cells and low viral loads.

In general, people don't think about suicide too often. Most people are familiar with the term *physician-assisted suicide*, where a trained doctor provides a patient the tools needed to commit suicide. In these cases, a terminally ill patient then takes action to end his or her own life, usually to alleviate intense physical pain that comes with certain conditions or diseases.

For people with end-stage AIDS, physician-assisted suicide is a consideration. For people who are testing positive now, occasional suicidal fantasies may be a way to cope, or a rare thought now and then. My favorite suicide fantasy is being hit by a bus. People always told me that "everyone is going to die someday; I could get hit by a bus tomorrow." I should be so lucky.

Don't worry about suicidal thoughts until you start working out the details of your plan. If you find yourself planning for something, you are not in your best frame of mind. Think about it: if the better option is to kill yourself, you are beyond miserable. And if you feel that bad, let someone help you. Talk to someone.

You might not believe it now, but relief is possible. It might come in the form of talking with another person, taking medicine, or spiritual belief. But if you're not receptive to the idea that things can get better, you'll have a harder time finding relief.

Suicide Hotline

FOR CRISIS CALLS: (800) 784-2433

IN A SENTENCE:

Anxiety, depression, and fleeting thoughts of suicide are common and normal, but planning suicide is a serious sign that you need help.

learning

Beating Anxiety and Depression

ANXIETY AND depression are the most common reasons that people with HIV seek assistance with mental health. The two conditions are different, but related. They can occur independently of each other at different times, or together at once. You can have depression with occasional periods of anxiety. On the other hand, you could be experiencing anxiety with occasional bouts of depression. Some treatments help both depression and anxiety at the same time.

If you suspect that depression or anxiety may be an issue for you, chances are that you will do one of the following:

○ do nothing and hope the conditions resolve
○ try behavior modification techniques such as regular exercise, yoga, or meditation
○ explore herbal supplements (not recommended if you're taking any other HIV medicine)
○ pursue psychotherapy (talking with a trained mental health professional)
○ try prescription medications
○ combine several of these approaches

Doing nothing is one option

Doing nothing for anxiety or depression is certainly an option that many people choose. Sure, you can pull the sheets over your head and hope for the best. Sometimes, clinical depression can lift on its own in six to twelve months. Sometimes, anxiety lessens with time as you become adjusted to living with HIV. But if these conditions turn severe or persist for extended periods of time, doing nothing will make things worse. Major depression in people with HIV is associated with decreased survival, increased hospital stays, and impaired quality of life. And 15 percent of depressed people take their own lives.

Exercise, yoga, or meditation can help

Exercise, yoga, and meditation might help—and can't hurt—in combating depression and anxiety. Research has shown exercise can have a positive impact on depression. You should already know this: Moving your body is good for your health. It's clearly documented that regular exercise improves depression. But you don't need science to tell you that exercise improves your mood. Some people swear by yoga as a way to battle anxiety. They say that by focusing on stretching and attaining the postures, you can tune out persistent or negative thoughts. Meditation may work in a similar way.

Herbal supplements may help with some conditions

Herbal supplements to treat anxiety and depression are controversial. Still, two-thirds of people with HIV use some form of alternative medicine. Many people don't tell their doctor that they are experimenting with herbs. If you're not currently taking HIV medicine or other medications, there's much less potential harm from herbal supplements

Psychotherapy (talk therapy) and support groups can keep you sane

Talking with other people has kept me from losing my marbles during my twenty years of having HIV. Let me be clear about this; what's kept me sane over the years has been talking with other people in a structured and therapeutic environment. By "structured and therapeutic," I mean a setting with some ground rules and a sense of purpose. Chatting with friends or family about your concerns does not always fall into this category (and, is sometimes counterproductive).

Talk therapy can take place in a group setting or one on one. Group settings can range from highly structured to very informal. For example, many AIDS organizations offer structured group therapy for people with HIV. The groups are usually limited in number, anywhere from five to 12 people per group. The groups usually meet once a week over the course of several weeks. They are usually headed by a trained professional who helps guide the conversation and enforces ground rules.

For me, group therapy was a lifesaver. At first I felt awkward about sharing my feelings with strangers. As I learned more about others in the group, I eventually got more comfortable. I felt less alone with my problems. In fact, other people in the group often described exactly what I was going through. Sometimes, they offered solutions that hadn't occurred to me. I didn't like everyone in the group—some I even despised. At times, group therapy seemed corny, melodramatic, and even depressing. Still, the groups eased my anxiety and fear about HIV.

Finding a therapist can make you crazy

One-on-one talk therapy, also called **psychotherapy** or counseling, is a whole different thing. When you seek out mental health care, you'll find a lot of confusing choices. Some of those choices may be limited by what you can afford, what your insurance covers, or what kind of access you have to health organizations. There's a list of resources at the end of this book to help you get started.

Mental health professionals who offer one-on-one talk therapy are often called "therapists" but this is an umbrella term that refers to a range of services. There are many types of licensed and unlicensed mental health professionals. They differ in educational backgrounds, training, state licensing, philosophy, and technique.

In the same way that you should interview potential new doctors, you should also interview therapists about their experience and training. You'll do best if you find someone with whom you share some values or experiences. The next step is figuring out if the mental health professional has experience with the type of problems you're having. Experience with HIV is a good idea. Some therapists offer a free initial consultation by phone or in person to help assess if they're right for you.

Here's a brief overview of the types of mental health professionals, their education, licenses, and certifications:

- ○ **Psychiatrists** are medical doctors, and can prescribe medication. Very few psychiatrists provide psychotherapy, but usually refer you to a psychotherapist. If you need medication, you will usually have to see a psychiatrist.
- ○ **Psychologists** usually have a doctorate degree and have completed an internship under supervision.
- ○ **Counselors** usually have a master's degree in counseling and have completed an internship under supervision, but not always. Counselors usually specialize in specific areas such as substance abuse, anxiety, or short-term crises.
- ○ **Clinical social workers** typically have a master's degree in social work and have completed a supervised internship.

ACADEMIC DEGREES:
M.A.—Master of Arts
M.S.—Master of Science
M.S.W.—Master of Social Work
Ph.D.—Doctor of Philosophy
Ed.D.—Doctor of Education
Psy.D.—Doctor of Psychology
M.Ed –Master of Educational Psychology
M.D.—Doctor of Medicine

LICENSES AND CERTIFICATIONS:
C.A.C.—Certified Addictions Counselor
C.S.W.—Certified Social Worker
C.S.W.—Clinical Social Worker
L.L.P.—Limited License Psychologist
L.P.—Licensed Psychologist
L.P.C.—Licensed Professional Counselor
L.M.F.T.—Licensed Marriage and Family Therapist
S.W.—Social Worker
P.C.C. or L.P.C.C.—Professional Clinical Counselors
C.P.C.—Certified Professional Counselor

The therapist-patient relationship may reflect other relationships

The weird thing about therapy is that the relationship between you and your therapist often reflects the relationships you have with other people in your life. For example, you might find a therapist with whom you're initially comfortable. But with time, you might start avoiding certain topics or missing appointments. You may even think you have good reasons for avoiding issues or missing sessions. What might be happening, however, is that you're uncomfortable with intimate relationships or afraid of being yourself. It may turn out that you're having the same problems with other people in your life.

On the other hand, you might get hooked up with a therapist who genuinely doesn't share your values or experiences. You might disagree about philosophical, social, cultural, or sexual issues. You are the only person who can determine if the therapist isn't right for you. I've certainly encountered therapists who've said or done things that disturbed me to the core. One therapist fell asleep on me in the middle of my session. Another said that I wasn't born "normal." In those cases, I knew the particular therapists weren't right for me.

At other points in my life, I had a great therapist who pushed me emotionally. This, too, was difficult—but in a good way. Often, I became angry at my therapist. Sometimes I resented the weekly appointment. Once, I failed to show up at all—for several weeks. But somehow I knew it wasn't the therapist; it was me being stubborn. When I stuck it out, when I continued to talk despite feeling uncomfortable, the payoff was worth the pain: I learned entirely new ways of seeing myself and the world around me.

Prescription drugs can help with mood disorders

In terms of depression, medicine has come a long way. The first generation of antidepressants was introduced in the 1950s. This class of drugs was dubbed **tricyclics** for their three-ringed molecular structure.

Although the trycyclics provide relief from depression, they were biochemically clumsy and produced severe side effects. Not much later came another class of drugs called **monoamine oxidase inhibitors** (**MAOIs**). Monoamine oxidase is an enzyme inside some nerves. Inhibition of this enzyme allows more norepinephrin, dopamine, and serotonin to be produced. Those three neurotransmitters are linked to moods and sleep. Decreased levels are associated with depressed moods.

The biggest problem with both types of these early antidepressants is their potential for serious side effects. MAOIs interact with certain foods to cause a sudden rise in blood pressure. Also, MAOIs sometimes produced tremors, insomnia, weight gain, and liver toxicity. Tricyclics can cause reduced mental acuity, drowsiness, dry mouth, blurred vision, weight gain, and sexual dysfunction.

Prozac-like drugs are effective in reducing depression

By the late 1980s, a third generation of antidepressants became available. The drugs, called selective serotonin reuptake inhibitors (SSRIs), have profound advantages over MAOIs and trycyclics. SSRIs are easier to tolerate because of their relative lack of unpleasant side effects, and they relieve depression about as effectively as the older medications. This new generation of antidepressants includes

- ○ citalopram (Celexa)
- ○ fluoxetine (Prozac)
- ○ paroxetine (Paxil)
- ○ sertraline (Zoloft)
- ○ fluvoxamine (Luvox)
- ○ escitalopram (Lexapro)

SSRIs are the most prescribed class of antidepressants. SSRIs have fewer interactions with other medications and are not associated with the weight gain common in people taking tricyclics. Also, SSRIs have a wide margin of safety in overdose and do not appear to be associated with withdrawal symptoms.

A relative of the SSRI family is a group of antidepressants called **partial serotonin reuptake inhibitors**. The mechanism of action for these related drugs is slightly different from standard SSRIs. In some cases, partial serotonin reuptake inhibitors may produce different side effects. These drugs include

- ○ venlafaxine (Effexor)
- ○ buspropian (Wellbutrin)

Anti-anxiety drugs can help you deal with panic

Symptoms of anxiety are relatively easy to treat with prescription drugs. These drugs are widely prescribed—and widely abused as well. If you're prone to substance abuse or are in recovery from drugs or alcohol, you should be careful about your intake of certain drugs used to treat anxiety. Certain classes of drugs may trigger a relapse or complicate the situation. In general, medications to treat anxiety are quite safe, have minimal side effects, and carry little danger of overdosing.

Benzodiazepines are the largest class of drugs used to treat anxiety. They work best if used for short periods of time to manage severe or occasional anxiety. The entire class of drugs may cause some "clouding" of the mind and "slowing" of motor skills. Some benzodiazepines stay in your body longer than others. Discuss with your doctor the risks and benefits of taking benzodiazepines, especially if you have addiction tendencies. The class of drugs includes:

- ○ lorazepam (Ativan and others)
- ○ alprazolam (Xanax)
- ○ clonazepam (Klonopin)
- ○ temazepam (Restoril)

Buspirone (BuSpar) is an alternative to the benzodiazepines. It is not sedating, has few mental side effects, and does not create dependency or addiction. Its major drawback is the long period before it takes effect, up to four weeks.

If you decide to pursue medication for anxiety or depression, it's a good idea to track any symptoms or any side effects from medication in your health journal. If, down the road, you and your doctor decide to switch or add medications, the details in your health journal can be especially useful.

IN A SENTENCE:

> *Anxiety and depression occur among people with HIV and there are several options for treating these conditions.*

Overcoming Nicotine, Marijuana, and Alcohol

AMONG HIV-POSITIVE people, non-HIV-related causes of death such as overdose, heart disease and cancer are on the rise. Nearly one in four people with HIV use illicit drugs and more than 12 percent are drug dependent—and that doesn't even count marijuana.

When you first smoke a cigarette, your intention isn't to get lung cancer. But when you smoke cigarettes over time, the odds of lung cancer increase dramatically. You wouldn't call a friend and say, "Let's meet at the bar for cirrhosis." Day by day, year after year, your choices add up. Each choice puts you on a road to either better health or worse health. In some cases, smoking crack or crystal meth will put you on a fast track to disaster. In other cases, it might be twenty years before smoking cigarettes catches up with you.

When it comes to substances, people generally use them for one of two reasons: They want to feel good or they want to feel better. Sensation seekers are looking for a novel or exciting experience, while the self-medicating types are attempting to escape life conditions, such as poverty or untreated mental disorders. They use substances as if they were treating themselves for anxiety or depression.

Whatever the initial reason, the vast majority of people abusing substances have a hard time quitting because their prolonged substance use changes the brain in fundamental and long-lasting ways. We've all know the drug burn-out stereotype.

While all illicit drugs have different effects on the brain, they also have a common bond: They trigger the release of dopamine, a brain chemical that is directly involved in the experience of pleasure. Feeling good about a job well done, getting pleasure from family or social interactions, feeling content, or feeling that one's life is meaningful all rely on dopamine. Drug addicts are addicted specifically to the meaningful dopamine spikes that drugs produce in the brain.

If you're indulging in excessive smoking, drinking, or drugs, you may be able to get control of your habits. But you may be deeper into addiction than you realize and may need professional help. If friends, coworkers, or family have noticed your substance abuse, then pay attention. They may be onto something.

Substances impair your thinking, which puts you at risk for more health problems, like wrapping your car around a tree. Substance abuse puts stress on the body, which is already burdened by HIV. Substance abuse reduces your chance of success with HIV treatment. But each day is a new day. At any point in your substance use, by examining your habits and learning about them, you can change directions and head to a healthier place.

Drug use is not a character flaw. The common notion of addiction-as-failure-of-character should be discarded. Instead, think of the strategies for stopping substance abuse just like the strategies for treating other chronic relapsing conditions like asthma or hypertension.

Quitting smoking seems impossible, but people do it all the time

If you have HIV, you're probably already a smoker. Like it or not, studies have shown that the type of people who smoke are the type of people who get HIV. In case you've been living under a rock, smoking causes a number of serious illnesses, from heart disease to cancer. Clearly, quitting smoking is a better choice for improved health. Tobacco and HIV—each on their own—can shorten your life.

If you have HIV and you smoke, you're more likely to develop the garden-variety problems associated with smoking. One recent study found that HIV-positive smokers were nearly eight times more likely to develop emphysema than smokers without the virus.

How to quit: nicotine replacement

NICOTINE REPLACEMENT therapy keeps the nicotine flowing, but without inhaling tobacco smoke. This gives you a chance to break the habit of smoking cigarettes. Down the road and when you're ready, you can wean yourself off the nicotine. Nicotine replacement comes in the form of a patch applied to the skin, several flavors of gum, lozenges (not as tasty as the gum, but still does the job), and inhalers that look and taste like real cigarettes. Nicotine replacement works best in the first days and months of quitting smoking.

Zyban and Wellbutrin are both the same drug–bupropion.

Some insurance companies don't cover Zyban, but they do cover Wellbutrin. They are the same drug called bupropion. Ask your doctor.

Chantix is a novel drug for nicotine addiction.

The FDA recently approved a new "molecular entity" with a generic name of varenicline tartrate (brand name: Chantix) to help cigarette smokers stop smoking. Chantix works by blocking nicotine from attaching to brain receptors.

Behavioral techniques and self-help groups produce better long-term outcomes by helping to change your thinking or shift your perspective, teaching your old brain a few new tricks. The combination of nicotine replacement and behavioral techniques are probably the best choice if you want to quit smoking for good.

Marijuana is a drug

Some people don't consider marijuana to be a true "drug." Whatever you consider marijuana to be, the real culprit in marijuana is tetrahydrocannabinol (THC). In the same way that nicotine is the addictive ingredient in tobacco, THC is the addictive ingredient in marijuana. THC is responsible for the "high" feeling that your brain learns to love so much. Is THC addictive? Maybe for you it is. It depends on your genes. According to NIDA, addiction is characterized by "compulsive, at times uncontrollable, drug craving, seeking, and use that persists even in the face of extremely negative consequences."

Smoking marijuana *excessively* causes a chemical irritation in the lungs, which can lead to bronchitis, says Daniel Berger, M.D. "Severe addiction problems with marijuana sometimes cause motivational aberrations. In other words, people are less motivated to do things for themselves that are consistent with good health practices. Marijuana smoking beyond moderation can have some consequences. But I don't perceive occasional marijuana use as being a problem."

Sometimes, marijuana is contaminated with insecticides, pesticides, fungus, and bacteria. Some HIV doctors suggest microwaving marijuana for ten to thirty seconds, especially to kill a fungus called *aspergillosis*.

Ecstasy is a psychedelic amphetamine

Ecstasy, or methylenedioxymethamphetamine (MDMA), is part hallucinogen and part stimulant. Ecstasy has LSD-like properties but it's more closely related to amphetamines. In high doses, Ecstasy can cause a sharp increase in body temperature, leading to muscle breakdown and kidney and heart failure. You might feel muscle tension and start to grind your teeth. You might feel nausea, experience blurred vision, or suffer from rapid eye movement, faintness, and chills or sweating. The drug also destroys serotonin-producing cells in the brain—not a good thing if you're prone to depression or anxiety.

A WORD OF CAUTION

Hepatically metabolized is a way of saying that your liver filters your blood. If you take too many drugs that are hepatically metabolized, your liver can't work fast enough. With this a backlog of drugs to be filtered, there's more drug in your blood.

On one hand, this is good news. One particular HIV drug, called ritonavir, is prescribed specifically to clog up the filters in your liver. Think of a fish tank with a broken filter. Just like algae builds up in a fish tank, the levels of all drugs in the blood can rise. This is often called ritonavir-boosted therapy.

On the other hand, too many hepatically metabolized drugs can lead to overdose. Doctors learned about ritonavir's properties by accident after an HIV patient on ritonavir also took Ecstasy. Because ritonavir clogs the liver, levels of the drug Ecstasy increased to deadly levels.

Alcohol use is common among people with HIV

Alcohol dependence rates for both men and women with HIV substantially exceed those in the general population. Some say that between 30 and 70 percent of people with HIV are dependent on alcohol. Men are especially at risk. Sure, booze is legal, but it doesn't mean it's good for your health. Heavy alcohol directly assaults your liver—and after a few years, especially with HIV treatment—the damage to your life can add up.

If you also happen to have chronic hepatitis C or hepatitis B, drinking any alcohol will speed the pace of liver damage. Light-to-moderate use can lead you to behave in ways that may be further damaging to your health. Having HIV doesn't rule out the possibility of a car crash.

If you're considering HIV medicine—or are already taking HIV medicine—you should know that alcohol reduces your chances of success over the long haul. Why? Alcohol use has a bad effect on:

○ metabolism of HIV drugs (alcohol changes the way your body absorbs the medicine)
○ adherence (you might choose to drink instead of taking your meds)
○ the balance between the virus and the immune system (to some degree, drinking does have a negative effect on your T-cells and viral load)

"The message to the physician and to the patients is to be aware that this can be very insidious," says Anthony S. Fauci, M.D., director of the National Institute of Allergy and Infectious Diseases. "It would really be a shame, that after all one has been through—finally getting your viral load down to below detectable levels, getting your hepatitis under control, being tested for cervical cancer or anal carcinoma from HPV—after all that, you end up knocking yourself out with chronic liver disease because you're drinking too much. Again, it's part of the whole health picture."

New medicine is available for alcohol withdrawal

Depending on your level of drinking, you might consider medications. Most drug addiction treatment programs also encourage people to participate in a self-help group during and after formal treatment. Some medications include:

CAMPRAL IS A NEW DRUG FOR ALCOHOLISM
Campral is the brand name of *acamprosate calcium,* a prescription medication that gained approval in the United States for the treatment of alcoholism. Thought to restore the normal brain balance in alcoholics, the drug helps reduce the physical distress and emotional discomfort (e.g. sweating, anxiety, sleep disturbances) associated with staying alcohol-free.

NALTREXONE IS ONE POSSIBILITY
Naltrexone is a medicine used primarily in the management of alcohol dependence and opioid addiction. Brand names include Revia and Vivitrol. In the past, low-dose naltrexone was used off-label as an experimental treat-

ment for certain immunological disorders. Its use in alcohol addiction has been studied and has been shown to be somewhat effective.

Antabuse is another option

Antabuse, the trade name for the drug tetraethylthiuram disulfide, alters the metabolism of alcohol in the body, making it impossible for you to get drunk without experiencing severe discomfort, such as vomiting.

Support groups can help with dopamine-based addictions

It doesn't matter if it's alcohol, marijuana, cocaine, gambling, or sex, you will eventually reach an equilibrium with your addictions. For some people, that means stopping the addiction altogether. Other people might just grow out of a bad phase, while other people reach equilibrium by incarceration, insanity, or death.

Understanding your addiction is a good first step. One place to do this is any 12-step meeting. What's the worst that can happen? You go into a room full of people who have something in common with you: they can't control their behavior. You all sit in a room and talk about your experiences with your behavior. Then someone will discuss the Twelve Steps to recovery. The format varies; often there's one speaker, but other times everyone takes a turn speaking.

In the United States and Europe, there are meetings everywhere. Many larger cities provide telephone numbers to call for specific times and locations. The best-known group is Alcoholics Anonymous (AA). AA is a huge, worldwide social network of recovered and recovering alcoholics. It involves a 12-step approach for recovering from alcoholism, but the philosophy is not specific to alcohol. The AA model has spawned related recovery programs including:

- Crystal Meth Anonymous (CMA)
- Narcotics Anonymous (NA)
- Cocaine Anonymous (CA)
- Sexual Compulsives Anonymous (SCA)
- Overeaters Anonymous (OA)
- Gambler's Anonymous (GA)

Some AA meetings in large cities may deal specifically with HIV and addiction. Although in some 12-step meetings, discussion of HIV is frowned upon—except at the specific meetings that deal directly with HIV issues. "I tried to go to 12-step meetings and share about HIV when I first got clean, but they told me it was an 'outside issue'," says Rosetta M. who is HIV-positive and a recovering addict. "Underneath it all, I think that there are people with HIV in the [AA and other 12-step] rooms and they are not sharing about it, so they resent when somebody comes in and shares about HIV. Or, they are still engaging in [risk] behaviors and they don't want you to rain on their parade. I think there's a lot of reasons and a lot of environments that people don't want to hear about HIV."

Still, 12-step approaches are often helpful for some people. You can find a 12-step meeting almost anytime or anywhere—if you know where to look. And if you can hook into one 12-step meeting, you can hook into a much bigger and better network of people who can help you. In the United States, there are meetings in every state and every major city. Many larger cities provide telephone numbers to call for specific times and locations. To find out more information about 12-step meetings, try calling an AIDS service organization, a state HIV hotline, or look online.

You know you're hooked when . . .

- ◯ A hit of this and a drink at one time was enough to hit the spot. These days, however, you crave two or three hits of this and maybe a six-pack of that.
- ◯ You drink to ease your hangover. Have you ever joked about having "a hair of the dog that bit you"?
- ◯ You run short of substances sooner than you planned. You could swear you just refilled that prescription for tranquilizers and already they're gone.
- ◯ You try to quit or cut down and it never seems to work out.
- ◯ You spend a lot of time waiting for your dealer friend or driving across town for God-knows-what.
- ◯ All your friends are the ones who really have addiction issues.
- ◯ You know it's a problem, but you just keep doing it.

IN A SENTENCE:

> *Drinking and smoking are dopamine-based behaviors that—with work on your part—can be overcome.*

learning

Understanding Cocaine, Heroin, and Prescription Drug Abuse

LIKE IT or not, if you're newly diagnosed with HIV, you must pay attention to your health. For many people, substance abuse gets in the way of good health. If you haven't picked up substance-abuse habits, a smart choice is never to start. If you think you can manage a cocaine or heroin habit, be assured it's only temporary. Three months or three years, it's just a matter of time until those addictions catch up to you.

A smart approach to cocaine use is not to begin in the first place

What makes crack cocaine distinct from powder cocaine is the delivery system. When you snort a line, your brain recognizes the drug slowly, over maybe ten to thirty minutes. The dopamine peak lasts around ten minutes. Then the rush dissipates almost entirely after about an hour.

But smoke a hit of crack and wham. It hits your brain like a brick. Peak dopamine levels max out in the first few seconds, lasting maybe one minute. So when you compare powder cocaine to crack cocaine, it's like condensing ten to thirty minutes dopamine experience into about one minute.

The problem is that one minute. The extreme dopamine spike alters the circuits in your brain in a way that makes you want more and more. It quickly distorts your perception of reality. Even with moderate use, crack can cause chest pain because cocaine puts stress on your heart. One recent study showed angiotensin converting enzyme (ACE) inhibitors might be helpful in people with cocaine addiction.

On the horizon is a new cocaine vaccine. A company called Xenova is developing this therapeutic vaccine, TA-CD, for the treatment of cocaine dependence. The vaccine does not stop the craving for cocaine, but will stop you from experiencing a high from cocaine. Some people might welcome this approach, others might not.

Valium and Xanax are benzodiazepines

Doctors often prescribe "benzos" for insomnia and anxiety. Chemically speaking, benzos cause anything from slight impairment to hypnosis. They're often called sedatives or tranquilizers. Most people don't notice benzo addiction until they're well into their habit. Discontinuing prolonged use of high-dose benzodiazepines can lead to serious withdrawal symptoms because all benzos work by slowing the brain's wiring. So when you quit, your brain's activity can rebound to the point of causing a seizure. If you're thinking about stopping your benzos, you should seek medical help beforehand.

Benzodiazepines come in a variety of shapes and colors. The most popular way to get the drug is by prescription. The benzodiazepines are a big family and they differ somewhat in side effects, potencies, timing, and the tendency to cause withdrawal. Drugs in the benzodiazepines family include:

- alprazolam (Xanax)
- lorazepam (Ativan)
- clonazepam (Klonopin)
- diazepam (Valium)
- oxazepam (Serax)
- temazepam (Restoril)
- flurazepam (Dalmane)
- triazolam (Halcion)

Heroin has a long history

A derivative of morphine, heroin's real name is diacetylmorphine. Heroin is the name that the Bayer Company gave to the drug in 1898. At the time, the drug was a blockbuster like today's Viagra. It took years for the medical profession to figure out the dangers of heroin addiction. Over time, the drug fell out of favor as "medicine" and became popular as a "drug."

Heroin is chemically created from morphine, a naturally occurring substance extracted from the seeds of certain poppy plants. Morphine is a member of a class of drugs also called opiates or narcotics. Other members of this class include hydrocodone (Vicodin) and codeine (Tylenol with Codeine).

- Heroin is typically sold as a white or brownish powder or as the black, sticky substance called "black tar heroin."
- It is usually injected, snorted, or smoked.
- Intravenous injection provides the greatest intensity and most rapid onset of euphoria (seven to eight seconds).
- Intramuscular injection produces a relatively slow onset of euphoria (five to eight minutes).
- Sniffed or smoked, peak effects are usually felt within ten to fifteen minutes.
- All three forms of heroin administration are addictive.

METHADONE IS A REPLACEMENT FOR HEROIN

Methodone treatment is to heroin addiction as nicotine replacement is to smoking cigarettes. Called *agonist maintenance treatment*, the methadone replaces the addicting opiate. This is mostly done in outpatient settings called methadone treatment programs. These programs use synthetic opiate medication, usually methadone or levomethadyl, given by mouth to prevent opiate withdrawal. These drugs block the effects of illicit opiate use, and decrease opiate craving. Patients stabilized on methadone or levomethadyl can function normally.

People stabilized on opiate agonists are better able to participate in counseling and other behavioral interventions. The best, most effective opiate agonist maintenance programs include individual and/or group counseling along with other needed medical, psychological, and social services.

Buprenorphine is an alternative to methadone

Buprenorphine is an alternative to methadone for treating opiate addiction. Buprenorphine is a partial opioid agonist. At low doses, it behaves as an agonist, and at high doses, as either an agonist or antagonist, depending on the circumstances. In 2002, buprenorphine hydrochloride (Subutex) was approved in the U.S. for the treatment of opioid dependence and is available by prescription.

Naltrexone is an alternative to buprenorphine

A drug called naltrexone is one drug used as "antagonist treatment," which blocks all the euphoria and effects of self-administered opiates. Because narcotic antagonists don't let you get "high" from opiates, it's hoped that the compulsion to use will be decreased. Naltrexone is also used to help treat alcoholism.

Principles of effective addiction treatment

The ultimate goal of all substance addiction treatment is to help to achieve lasting abstinence. Immediate goals are to (1) reduce your drug use, (2) improve your functioning, and (3) minimize medical and social complications.

According to the National Institute on Drug Abuse, drug addiction treatment should include the following principles.

- No single treatment is appropriate for all individuals. You and your genes are unique. What works for the guy down the street might not work for you.
- Treatment needs to be easily available. You might change your mind if you find treatment is a hassle.
- Treatment should help all of you, not just your drug use. You might need assistance with medical, psychological, social, vocational, or legal issues.
- Assess often and modify when necessary. Your doctor might try varying combinations of services and treatment components during the course of treatment and recovery.
- Give addiction treatment time to work. Research suggests that a minimum of three months is needed for most. People usually leave treatment prematurely.

○ Individual and/or group counseling is critical. In counseling, you discuss motivation, tricks to resist drugs, replacing drug activities with nondrug activities.

○ Medications are an important element of treatment. Medications such as methadone and levomethadyl (also known as LAAM) are effective in helping people who are addicted to heroin or other opiates. Naltrexone is also an effective medication for some opiate addicts and some patients with co-occurring alcohol dependence.

○ Treat addiction and coexisting mood disorders in an integrated way. Your doctor should assess you for other mood disorders such as anxiety or depression.

○ Medical detoxification is only the first stage of addiction treatment. Detox alone is rarely sufficient to help addicts achieve long-term abstinence.

○ Treatment does not need to be voluntary to be effective. You might need to be forced into treatment.

○ Possible drug use during treatment is a concern. Urinalysis and other tests can help you withstand urges to use lapse.

○ Address HIV and hepatitis C in addiction treatment. Counseling also can help you manage your health better.

○ Recovery from drug addiction is a long-term process, often with relapses. Don't get discouraged if you relapse a few times.

IN A SENTENCE:

There are clear options to recover from cocaine, heroin, and other addictions.

Crystal Meth: Fast Track to Disaster

OUTSIDE STARBUCKS, I'm sitting and talking on my cell when I notice someone crossing the street. He's a well-dressed young guy and he's brazenly stepping off the curb without regard to passing cars. He's puffing out his chest, arms slightly curled like a posing weightlifter. As he reaches my side of the street, I notice he's jutting out his lower jaw, then clenching it. He stops for a moment and aggressively scans the crowd outside the coffee shop. He zeroes in on me, saunters over, and fake smiles, while also grinding his teeth. He looks sweaty. I recognize him as tweaker.

"Hey," he says. "Can I have some money?"

When I tell him no, he moves his attention to someone else.

A *tweaker* is a person who uses crystal meth. The good news is that, in general, crystal meth abuse is down somewhat in the general population. The bad news, however, is that crystal meth abuse continues to be particular problem among men who have sex with men.

As a chemical, crystal meth is especially good at tricking your brain into feeling really good. Specifically, the drug stimulates the part of your brain that controls your sense of pleasure and reward. This stimulation happens faster than with most other drugs. Meth is cheap, it lasts a long time, and it makes you feel good—at least at first.

The problem is that your brain want more and more drug-induced pleasure. Your brain rewires itself so that it begins to need the drug. It wants to recreate those first feel-good moments, so it tells you to go out and get more meth. It's the reason why, waiting at a traffic light, you suddenly think about using crystal.

The other complication is that meth distorts the way you see reality. Although if you use meth, you might not think that's true. The young guy who recklessly crossed the street and asked me for money, I can't say what he was thinking. But I know he wasn't seeing the same reality as the rest of us at Starbucks.

We know people with HIV are likely to use crystal meth HIV or not, the story is the same for everyone: Meth use starts good and ends bad. Period. I have not heard one story about tweakers getting job promotions. Or achieving their goals. Or find even finding peace of mind. Instead, you hear cliché stories about decline and despair. That's where meth goes. It might take three months or three years, but that's where the road of meth leads.

If you're newly diagnosed with HIV, using meth is not a path for either health or happiness. If you haven't used the drug, a smart choice is never to start (and that's not just anti-drug propaganda). First time use is always a choice.

All meth users start off as casual users

Jeff W. first tried meth after he was laid off from his dot-com job. Only months earlier, he got the news about having HIV. "When I first realized I was positive, I was paranoid to let anyone know. I'm in the closet about being positive. I became afraid of even going to see a doctor because people might see me walking in the clinic. Then taking HIV meds, they became a reminder. So I stopped taking them. I just wanted to forget about it."

Jeff W. started using crystal meth with friends, hanging out at clubs and bars. "Here's some powder in a bottle. Just snort a couple bumps. It'll help you stay up." For Jeff W., the first time was one bump. Then another. Then it was three bumps.

"People want to forget about the fact that they're HIV positive," says Daniel Berger, M.D., an HIV specialist in Chicago. "People want to go out and have a good time and not have to confront their disease. They want to have normal sex lives. When they're in a normal state of mental being, they feel like they can't have a normal sex life. They just can't relax or enjoy themselves. It's only when they get high that they can forget. It's almost a reflexive activity to find ways to forget about your HIV status."

If there's anything that can make you forget about HIV, it's crystal meth. On it, people often feel energetic, alert, talkative, or sexually aroused. It's long name is methamphetamine, while goes by slang names such as speed, crank, crystal, tina, or ice. Sometimes it looks like small chips of ice. Other times it looks more like salt. It's basically odorless and tastes bitter. It can be snorted, absorbed by mucous membranes, smoked, or injected into a vein. Immediately, it excites your nervous system, which increases your heart rate and breathing. You lose your appetite. Your body heats up.

People respond to chemicals in different ways. Not all brains are built the same way. For example, if you were born with particular addiction genes, then drinking alcohol might feel great. But if you weren't born with these genes, then drinking alcohol might feel good—but not great. It's the same story for food, sex, drugs, gambling, or anything else related to immediate pleasure. It depends on your genes and what you encounter in life.

Crystal meth is the ingredient for party and play

The whole scene is seductive, says Cyril Gaultier, M.D, an infectious disease and HIV specialist in Palm Springs, California. He sees a large number of HIV patients. "Again and again I've heard stories that, 'Wow! It made me feel so good. I was thinking so clearly. I was on top of the world. I was very popular. I felt so sexy. I had the best sex of my life.'"

Meth users report that the drug lowers social inhibition. It makes it easier to break the ice and interact with other people. "It's a very sexual drug," says Jeff W. "You feel horny and you become fixated about whatever you're doing. And the other person's high too. You figure they're high, so they won't be as critical about you and what's going on. Since you care less, I care less. We can be together."

The crystal meth high eventually turns bad

Meth leads to a distortion of reality faster than with most other illicit drugs. When meth users are high, they don't see their behavior as being altered. In fact, it's just the opposite: they think they see things quite clearly.

At least improve your odds

If you're going to use crystal meth, at least take some precautions. Steven J. Lee, M.D., is the author of *Overcoming Crystal Meth Addiction–The Essential Guide to Getting Clean*. Lee is a private practice physician in New York City who specializes in addiction psychiatry. He offers some important reminders:

○ If you are doing bumps or snorting lines, never share straws, rolled-up dollar bills, keys, or "bullets." Always use your own. Sharing these snorting tools increases the risk of catching or transmitting HIV, hepatitis B and C, and other illnesses.

○ If you slam, don't share needles. If you must share, clean your needles with bleach and water before the next user's turn.

○ Pace yourself.

○ Take a break every hour to rest and hydrate. Drink liquids with sugar and electrolytes, such as fruit juices or Gatorade.

○ Fluids are important for oral health. "Meth mouth" results from long-term crystal use is characterized by softened, misshaped, and decayed teeth and bleeding, infected gums.

○ If you grind your teeth, or clench your jaw when you're high, try chewing sugar-free gum. Try chewing a gum like Biotene, which promotes saliva secretion.

Dr. Berger offers a few more tips for people with HIV:

○ Don't mix crystal meth with other drugs.

○ Afterward, get plenty of rest.

○ If you're taking HIV meds, take your HIV meds on schedule.

○ Stay monitored by a physician.

○ Practice safe sex.

"They believe that they feel so good, they don't perceive there being a reason to stop using," says Dr. Berger, "even as they get into trouble." In other words, they start missing out on friendships, they don't socialize, they miss work, ignore their bills, start getting into debt. As this continues, many users fail to perceive a problem and continue using.

Meth users tend to bond together and not always for the better. For instance, as Jeff W.'s meth use escalated, he lost his job, and money became tight. His solution? His drug dealer moved into his house to help pay the mortgage. "I really thought he was my friend," says Jeff W.

Other acquaintances were people not at their best. "You meet people who are already messed up, people who are paranoid and shaky. They only come over to use up your stuff. People steal; they steal your drugs, they steal your money, they steal your DVD player, or whatever."

What's too much? According to Dr. Berger, the key is really knowing how much and how often you use crystal meth. Have you missed work because of it? How much time do you spend recuperating from a run on the drug?

"Maybe twice a month is where some people haven't totally lost their sense of reality, where they can actually undergo a self-examination and look at themselves and try to get some help."

Crystal meth changes the brain. And so individuals often develop cognitive dysfunction problems. They often develop psychological problems that are sometimes irreversible. Even after some individuals do manage to quit or stop using, they're left with long-term psychological consequences.

As for physical consequences, Berger sees these in his medical practice on a daily basis. He notes that crystal is often cut with various chemicals, such as bleach, antifreeze, battery acid, lantern fuel, or drain cleaner. These chemicals destroy the integrity of skin and mucous tissues. This damage of body tissues is a portal for other infections and complications.

The complications can include bacterial infections that manifest as boils or abscesses anywhere on the body. "I've seen them occur on their face, chest, extremities, back, buttocks, around their rectum and genitals," says Berger. "Treatment for this often requires IV antibiotics and it's life threatening."

IN A SENTENCE:

> *Crystal meth use starts good and always ends bad.*

learning

Leaving Crystal Meth

BRIAN RISLEY is a counselor at AIDS Project Los Angeles (APLA). Years ago, long before his Lead Treatment Educator position at APLA, Risley launched a support group for people who were newly diagnosed with HIV. Every Wednesday for ten years, his support group has discussed issues and problems facing the newly diagnosed. The group is a microcosm of the larger population of people with HIV. The group meets every Wednesday in Hollywood, California. He's certainly seen the effect of what's going on out there with crystal meth.

His advice: First recognize that you have problem. Then say "I need help." Once you start telling yourself *and* other people that you need help with crystal meth and HIV, you can easily plug into a bigger and better network of people.

Step one is asking another person for help

If you are ready to quit using crystal meth, Risley offers a few practical tips for plugging into a better network of people:

- Ask for help from a friend who's already in a 12-step program. You two can attend a meeting and then you'll hear about other resources. Or you'll see something posted on bulletin board.
- Go online and investigate your options.

- If you have insurance, call your health plan and describe the type of mental health professional you want. "Sometimes, when you call, you get a call back from a therapist in the network who's exactly what you don't want. So even when you have insurance with a network and they do an 'intake,' it might not fit."
- If you have insurance, consider going directly into a rehab facility. "And once you go to a rehab facility, that opens a whole bunch of doors for you."
- Find an AIDS service organization that has a good reputation. If you come to APLA, we have licensed therapists on staff. "It's plugging into initial care and hopefully getting a referral from somebody. Getting a referral from your doctor is probably the best resource, or coming to a place like APLA."
- If you don't have insurance you can't always go to a county facility. Sometimes there are beds available for someone without insurance. "I'm always concerned about that person who doesn't have insurance. Someone with insurance is always going to be better off."

In most major cities, there is some organization or clinic that provides services, direct medical, as well as mental health services. Most major cities have some organization where you can ask for help.

Rehab and detox are the first steps to meth recovery

Addiction research has come a long way in the last 20 years. Research shows that combining addiction medicine with behavioral—talk therapy—tends to produce the best results. In some cases, people may need to "take a vacation" from their regular routine and check into a structured environment. Most people call this *drug rehabilitation, drug rehab* or just *rehab*. One of the first goals of rehab is to cut off the supply the addictive substance in a process called *detoxification,* or just *detox*.

Detox works best under the care of a physician in a medical setting—either in-patient or out-patient. It eases physical symptoms directly related to stopping the addictive substance. Withdrawal can be dangerous or fatal. Doctors sometimes use medicine when "detoxing" a patient from opiates, nicotine, benzodiazepines, alcohol, and barbiturates. Unfortunately, there are no specific drugs approved the FDA for treating meth addiction.

One company called Hythiam is studying the usefulness of three older, FDA-approved medicines together to reduce symptoms of methamphetamine withdrawal. The company has branded the name Prometa to represent a "treatment protocol designed to correct the long-term physiological effects induced by repeated exposure to methamphetamine." The University of California, Los Angeles is conducting a clinical trial to assess the efficacy of the Prometa when it's compared to a placebo.

According to the *Los Angeles Times,* Prometa involves administering an intravenous (IV) medicine called flumazenil and two oral drugs: gabapentin and hydroxyzine. These drugs are administered in an outpatient setting. The chemical compounds called *flumazenil, gabapentin,* and *hydroxyzine* are not approved by the U.S. by the Food and Drug Administration (FDA) for the treatment of addiction.

Flumazenil is an antidote for benzo overdose

Flumazenil is a benzodiazepine (or benzo) antagonist, which means that it counteracts the effects of certain sedatives such Valium or Xanax. It's mainly administered by IV in hospitals as an antidote for benzodiazepine overdose. Other names include Mazicon and Romazicon.

Gabapentin is a nerve drug called Neurontin

Gabapentin is the generic name of this chemical, while Neurontin is the brand name. Gabapentin is primarily used to relieve pain, especially nerve-related pain. Gabapentin was originally approved by the FDA to help control seizures. Later, it was approved for painful herpes-related outbreaks like shingles and painful peripheral neuropathies like those caused by HIV meds. The chemical is also used "off-label" for a variety of conditions. When used for pain, one patient described the drug as moderately helpful. "Mostly it made me feel like I was moving in slow motion. I'd think, 'move my foot' and then for what seemed like seconds later, my foot would move."

Hydroxyzine is a sedating antihistamine

Hydroxyzine is a chemical that is mostly used as an antihistamine to relieve or prevent allergy symptoms. Brand names include Atarax, Vistaril, Hyzine, Ucerax, and Serecid. Sometimes this chemical is used to control nausea and vomiting, including motion sickness. Other times it's used to reduce anxiety, sometimes associated with alcohol withdrawal. Basically, it's a sedating antihistamine.

Hythiam says that the intent of Prometa is to quiet cravings and improve mental clarity. After the initial treatment, a patient on the treatment protocol then receives one month of prescription medications and nutritional supplements. The company then encourages patients to seek some form of individual or group therapy.

Support groups can help with meth addiction

Meth use starts good and ends bad, period. Support groups are especially good for dealing with life's bad patches. "I think that peer support is valuable," says Risley. "Having a place to go to validate your feelings, a place where you're not isolating. That's important."

The best-known support group is Alcoholics Anonymous (AA). The twelve-step philosophy is not intrinsically related to alcohol. The AA model has spawned related recovery programs including Crystal Meth Anonymous and Narcotics Anonymous.

Trusted Web sites for addiction support and recovery:

www.aa.org

www.crystalmeth.org

www.tweaker.org

www.thoughtsonspeed.com

www.harmreduction.org

It takes work to stay on the road to recovery

Part of recovery is dealing with the underlying issues for substance abuse. Risley says that crystal meth addiction isn't just a hedonistic habit, it's a symptom of depression or low self-esteem. This was certainly the case with Jeff W., who's now clean for six months with the help of AA and CMA.

He relapsed once, but he knows he's on a better road. "It gave me inner content. I'd never felt comfortable in my own skin. I could probably still feel more comfortable, but I've never felt this content, or this inner peace. HIV is part of me. I'd rather not be positive, but since I am, so be it. And that's what I've been struggling trying to get."

With a clear and calm mind, Jeff W. confronts reality and deals with problems—and then takes action. For example, in terms of dealing with HIV he is now seeing a doctor regularly, taking HIV meds, and exercising. He goes to an AA or CMA meeting once a day. He's says that listening to other people's experiences is key.

IN A SENTENCE:

> *When you are ready to quit crystal meth, ask someone for help.*

Sex Addiction: What You Should Know

"HAVING SEX is not a bad thing." That's one of the first things that Jeffrey Parsons, Ph.D., says about sex and HIV. "In fact, people need healthy sex lives as part of a healthy life in general."

Parsons knows sex. He's a research psychologist and a professor of psychology at Hunter College of the City University of New York. He's also Director of the Center for HIV/AIDS Educational Studies and Training. His research focuses on HIV and sexual health, with a particular emphasis on sexual addiction and substance abuse, especially among people with HIV.

Researchers estimate that sexual addiction (also called *sexual compulsion*) exists in 3 to 6 percent of the total U.S. population. It occurs significantly more in men than in women. And among HIV-positive men who have sex with men, over 30 percent experience issues with sexual addiction.

While sexual addiction can wreak havoc on your life, there is some good news. Sexual addiction, like other addictions, can be overcome by a variety of methods, including talk therapy, self-help groups, and medications. But the first step is knowing if it's truly a problem.

Sexual addiction and compulsion are different names for the same thing

There's a fine line between addiction and compulsion. Addiction is a physical need for a particular substance, while compulsion is a desire to engage in a particular behavior. The zinger is that some behaviors trigger the brain to produce the same chemicals that are produced with substance addiction: dopamine. The biggest problem with dopamine is that it causes an addiction-like state in the brain. With enough spikes of dopamine over time, your brain depends on those spikes. And some brains are genetically prone to needing dopamine.

Having sex *and* thinking about sex both lead to dopamine spikes. But unlike a craving for drugs, a craving for sex can take the form of sexual fantasies and sexual behaviors. Both can interfere with your life. Some examples are:

○ Having more sex and with more partners than you had originally intended
○ Wanting to limit your sexual activity, but not being successful
○ Thinking about sex instead of thinking about other important things
○ Spending way too much time doing things related to sex, such as spending hours online cruising for partners or viewing porn
○ Neglecting your work, school, or family because you were pursuing sex
○ Engaging in sexual behavior despite negative consequences, such as broken relationships or potential health risks
○ Needing more and more sexual behavior over time
○ Feeling irritable when you can't engage in sexual behavior

The Society for the Advancement of Sexual Health says that fantasies or behaviors can spiral out of control. These out-of-control behaviors can get worse at times and improve other times. The organization offers three basic considerations if you're wondering if a particular behavior is out of control:

○ Have you lost control over *choosing* to engage in your out-of-control sexual behavior?
○ Are you experiencing significant consequences because of your out-of-control sexual behavior?
○ Are you constantly thinking about your out-of-control sexual behavior, even when you don't want to?

The tipping point is when your out-of-control sexual behavior causes stress or problems. "There are people who are fully capable of having sex on a daily basis, with multiple partners, with the use of pornography, and the use of Internet," says Parsons, "but they're having perfectly satisfying, functional lives. That's great.

"But when a person says 'I'll meet you for dinner on Friday night' and he doesn't show up because he can't leave the bathhouse, or when she gets fired from her job because a one-hour lunch turned into a three-hour tryst in the park," says Parsons, "the line has probably been crossed."

Are you a sex addict?

Researchers in the field of sexual health have developed a test that's used to assess tendencies toward sexual addiction. The Sexual Compulsivity Scale has been used in the general population and among people with HIV. In fact, one new study showed that the Sexual Compulsivity Scale is "reliable and valid in assessing men and women infected with HIV."

SEXUAL COMPULSIVITY SCALE

A number of statements that some people have used to describe themselves are given below. Read each statement and then circle the number to show how well you believe the statement describes you.

1 = Not at all
2 = Slightly
3 = Mainly
4 = Very Much

My sexual appetite has gotten in the way of my relationships.
   1   2   3   4

My sexual thoughts and behaviors are causing problems in my life.
   1   2   3   4

My desires to have sex have disrupted my daily life.
   1   2   3   4

I sometimes fail to meet my commitments and responsibilities because of my sexual behaviors.
   1   2   3   4

I sometimes get so horny I could lose control.

    1   2   3   4

I find myself thinking about sex while at work.

    1   2   3   4

I feel that sexual thoughts and feelings are stronger than I am.

    1   2   3   4

I have to struggle to control my sexual thoughts and behavior.

    1   2   3   4

I think about sex more than I would like to.

    1   2   3   4

It has been difficult for me to find sex partners who desire having sex as much as I want to.

    1   2   3   4

TO FIND OUT YOUR SCORE:

Add the numbers that you circled. Then, divide by number of circles. For example, if you added up all the numbers and got 16 (and you answered all 10 items), then you would divide 16 by 10. Your score would be 1.6.

WHAT YOUR SCORE MEANS:

Researchers generally agree that people who score 2.5 or above are "more addicted than not addicted." Being more addicted than not generally leads to problems. Also, according to researchers, it's more important to be comfortable with your own responses. Whatever your score, the Sexual Compulsivity Scale is only an initial screening test that can help some people identify sexual addiction problems. Ultimately, you must decide for yourself if sexual addiction is a problem.

There are many ways to deal with sex addiction

The first step in changing sexual behavior is deciding if it's truly a problem. The second step is taking action. While the best action depends upon your unique situation, there are many avenues to explore. While many people may think that abstinence is the key, Parsons notes, "To simply stop having sex isn't the most psychologically well-adjusted way to handle [sexually compulsive behavior]. But I think that there are times that sexual abstinence is appropriate."

If you are truly concerned about sex addiction, Parsons suggests seeking out a mental health professional who has training and experience in this area.

Unfortunately, many counselors and therapists don't see sexual addiction or compulsivity as a bona fide condition. However, one resource for locating a suitable health-care professional is the Society for the Advancement of Sexual Health (SASH), a nonprofit professional organization that helps those who suffer from out-of-control sexual behavior. SASH offers a Web site (www.sash.net) with a list of mental health providers around the country. Although SASH doesn't officially endorse any of its resources, the providers listed are both experienced and sensitive to the issues of sexual addiction.

Support groups work for some people

One popular support group is called Sexual Compulsive Anonymous (SCA). SCA is based on the 12-step model of Alcoholics Anonymous (AA), but instead of alcohol, the problem is compulsive behavior related to sex. SCA meetings are open to anyone who wants to recover from sexual compulsion, regardless of their gender or sexual orientations.

The main difference between SCA and AA is that while you can abstain from alcohol, abstaining from sex is not the answer for most. The focus of SCA is not to repress sexuality, but to help you express it in ways that don't steal your time and energy—or place you in legal jeopardy. Each member develops a sexual recovery plan, defining what sexual sobriety means for him or herself. Visit SCA's Web site, www.sca-recovery.org, for more information.

Over the years, various offshoots have grown. Some of the 12-step groups use slightly different language when they talk about sexual issues or behaviors. Other groups include more emotional aspect of sexual addiction. They include:

O   Sex and Love Addicts Anonymous
O   Sexual Compulsives Anonymous
O   Sex Addicts Anonymous
O   Sexaholics Anonymous

Parsons notes that 12-step groups can help decrease problem behaviors and provide support. "My feeling about 12-step groups is that they work very well for some people," he says. "It doesn't work at all for other people.

And still, for others, it's a good thing to have in addition to some other form of professional treatment."

Antidepressants may help with sexual addiction

One treatment option for sexual addiction is prescription medication that's generically called citalopram, but generally goes by the brand name of Celexa.

Citalopram is used to treat depression, body dysmorphic disorder, and anxiety. The drug belongs to a class of Prozac-like drugs known as selective serotonin reuptake inhibitors (SSRI)—the same class of drugs associated with sexual dysfunction. Still, one recent study found some effectiveness of citalopram for treating symptoms of sexual compulsion.

SSRIs are the most—prescribed class of antidepressants. This generation of antidepressants includes:

○ citalopram oxalate (Celexa)
○ escitalopram oxalate (Lexapro)
○ fluoxetine (Prozac)
○ fluvoxamine (Luvox)
○ paroxetine (Paxil)
○ sertraline (Zoloft)

Good news about sex, the Internet, and HIV

There's no shortage of articles and research about how the Internet fuels the spread of HIV. However, according to Parsons, the Internet is also an untapped tool for dowsing the virus as well.

One the biggest barriers to having safe sex is having to talk about safe sex. In the heat of the moment, when two people are naked, that's probably not the best time to negotiate safe sex rules. Sexual negotiation should happen well before that point of arousal—and that's why online communication can be effective. It allows people to disclose their HIV status while remaining anonymous.

"Sero-sorting" is what researchers call this online trend of HIV disclosure. For example, people are posting their HIV status online before they meet potential sex partners. Sometimes they use the term "clean" to mean HIV negative and "poz" to mean HIV positive. Of course, one in four people with

HIV don't know they have the virus. So, it's possible that someone may advertise themselves as "clean" when—unknown even to themselves—they're actually "poz."

Sero-sorting is happening online: people are specifically looking for other people of the same HIV status. Poz people are pairing up with other poz people. And when there's crossover, at least there's a potential for prior discussion. And the research is already clear that when sexual negotiation takes place in advance, it's more likely to be safer sex.

It's easy to demonize something like the Internet as a venue for HIV transmission. But Parsons imagines a day when sex addiction interventions will be online and available to anyone who needs them. "The Internet can be an incredibly beneficial tool in terms of HIV. It can also be a problem. It just depends on how people use it."

IN A SENTENCE:

> *If a sexual behavior is causing you problems—or preventing your progress—it's probably not a healthy sex life.*

learning

Eat to Lose Fat, Exercise to Gain Muscle

AMERICANS ARE getting fat and people with HIV are no different. Between 1991 and 2000, obesity among the general population increased by 60 percent, with one in five being obese and one in three being overweight. At the same time, almost one in four Americans with HIV are dieting to lose weight.

Half the Fat of Regular People
HIV population compared to the general population

GENERAL POPULATION
Two in three—overweight
Two in five—obese

PEOPLE WITH HIV
One in three—overweight
One in ten—obese

Being half as fat as the general population is not saying much. Clearly, the old image of people with HIV as being undernourished and emaciated no longer holds true. Since the introduction of the new HIV treatments, the prevalence of malnutrition among the HIV population has fallen by almost 50 percent. Even more encouraging is a 77 percent decrease in the prevalence of "wasting," a specific medical condition characterized by "unintentional loss of more than 10 percent of body weight." It's certainly no mistake that the decrease of wasting rates is almost identical to the decrease of rates of "full-blown" AIDS. The lesson: less AIDS, less wasting.

A recent study showed that the rates of wasting were still significant among people with HIV. However, the study also showed that the rates of obesity among the same population were more common than the rates of wasting:

○ 6 percent—wasting
○ 34 percent—overweight
○ 9 percent—obese

The researchers were careful to note that HIV treatment itself was not the cause of being overweight or obese. Instead, they concluded that "dietary and lifestyle advice" should be included as a component of HIV treatment.

At the same time, people who are taking HIV treatment are increasingly reporting that their levels of cholesterol and triglycerides, both of which are special types of fat found in the blood, are climbing. Cholesterol and triglycerides are associated with obesity, diabetes, high blood pressure, and heart problems—all of which are also being reported among people with HIV. (There's a related but somewhat different condition called **lipodystrophy**, which is discussed later in this book.)

What does all this mean for you? It means that having HIV doesn't get you off the hook when it comes to nutritious eating and honest exercise. In fact, healthy eating and exercise are very likely to be more important because you have the virus. Let's face it, if you plan on living a long time with HIV, you'll need to eat well and exercise.

Television, bookstores, magazine racks, and the Internet are brimming with the latest "news" on fitness and diet fads. Some of the advice is good, but most of it seems conflicting, confusing, and probably even misleading.

Don't let this noise distract you from the time-tested, proven, safe, and sound principles of fitness:

1. If you're below a healthy weight, you should eat nutritiously and exercise more often to gain or maintain weight.
2. If you're overweight, you should eat nutritiously in smaller portions and exercise more often to lose weight.

It really is that simple.

What "they" say about nutrition and HIV is wrong

Fortunately, it's a new ball game when it comes to HIV. Unfortunately, the conventional wisdom about nutrition for people with HIV is stuck in the 1990s. Doctors don't manage HIV like they did back then. In the same way, you shouldn't be eating like you're on death's door—unless, of course, your goal is to be on death's door.

If you've been to an HIV doctor or an HIV clinic, you've probably seen all the colorful brochures that claim wasting is still a major problem and that the latest pill or steroid can help you "gain weight." What these pharmaceutical-sponsored brochures fail to mention is that their claims are based on old research.

The advice offered by these brochures is based on research done in the 1990s. Back then, people with HIV were generally sicker, had higher viral loads and lower T-cells. At the time, the nutritional needs of these people were very different.

In the 1990s, treatments and a booming business emerged to help people with HIV combat the physical deterioration that's associated with AIDS. Pharmaceutical companies developed a variety of new products. Dieticians and physical therapists began selling their services to people with AIDS. Makers of nutritional and herbal supplements proliferated. "Crisis management" was the mantra of the times.

Today, however, the crisis is over and the focus should be on maintaining health for the long term. Look carefully at those brochures—they're ultimately trying to sell you something or "prime their market." There's a lot of money in the business of prescriptions or supplements to manipulate body weight.

Think about nutrition and HIV in one of two ways

There are new ways to think about HIV. On one hand, there's "uncontrolled HIV," which means that the virus is running rampant, gobbling up T-cells, and generally making a mess of your body. People with moderate-to-high viral load levels, depleted immune systems, or both, have uncontrolled HIV. This was the case with many people in the 1990s. On the other hand, there's "controlled HIV." In this state, HIV treatments are keeping the virus in check. People with controlled HIV have very low viral loads that may be below the limit of detection.

A critical distinction, however, is *how* the virus is being controlled. If you have a low viral load and you're not taking HIV medicine, it means your immune system is working double duty. For the purposes of nutrition, let's refer to that scenario as "uncontrolled HIV." If you are taking HIV medicine, and your viral load is very low or undetectable, that's controlled HIV. Your immune system doesn't need to work as hard, and your nutritional needs may change as well.

Imagine this: You're in a log cabin on a very cold night. To stay warm, you find some wood logs and stoke up a fire in the fireplace. The cabin warms up to a nice cozy temperature.

In this metaphor, think of the cabin as your body, the fireplace as your immune system, and the wood logs as the food you eat. In your cabin, you throw a log on the fire every few hours to keep the temperature comfortable, just as you would eat three times a day to remain healthy. This is the normal state of healthy human bodies.

Now imagine that someone throws a rock through a window in your cabin. This is a little like getting infected with HIV. Of course, the cabin may stay warm at first, but you know it won't last long because the heat is escaping through the window faster than the fireplace can make more heat. What do you do? You have two choices: start tossing more logs in the fireplace more often, or patch the window.

Back in the 1990s, people with HIV did not have the right treatments to "patch the hole in the window." So the obvious choice—back then— was to start throwing logs on the fire. At the time, researchers and nutritionists recommended that people with HIV eat more food, especially rich, fatty food to fuel their broken immune systems. After all, the virus and the immune system were battling fiercely. People with HIV ate up to provide the fuel, as food, for both the virus and the immune system. "Eat!" the researchers told people with HIV, sometimes suggesting they take in double the calories and protein. It made sense back then.

Now imagine you're back in the cabin with a broken window and you haven't gotten around to patching the window. Instead, you decide to burn logs more often to keep the heat at a comfortable level. But, you also know there's only a limited number of trees to burn and eventually you'll run short.

Finally, you decide it's time to patch the window. In this example, patching the window is like taking HIV medicine: You fix the underlying problem. However, after you fix the window, would you continue to throw logs on theire at the same rate? Of course not. The cabin would get too hot. In the same way, if you continue to eat as the researchers told the HIV-positive throughout the 1990s, you'd get fat and put yourself at other health risks such as heart disease and diabetes.

Diabetes and HIV

WHY PEOPLE with HIV should care about Type 2 diabetes:

○ Diabetes risk increased threefold in HIV-positive women treated with anti-HIV drugs called protease inhibitors.
○ Research has shown increases in the incidence of diabetes among HIV-positives, compared to HIV-negatives.
○ Among people with HIV, 34 percent are overweight and 9 percent are obese.
○ Weight gain of eleven to eighteen pounds doubles your risk of developing type 2 diabetes.
○ About 80 percent of people with diabetes are overweight or obese.
○ One-third of people with diabetes don't know that they have it.

WHAT IS DIABETES?

Diabetes is a disorder of metabolism—the way our bodies use digested food for growth and energy. Most of the food we eat gets converted into glucose, which is the body's main source of energy. Cells can only absorb glucose when insulin, a hormone made by the pancreas, is present.

When you have diabetes, you don't produce or respond to insulin. With diabetes, glucose builds up in the blood, overflows into the urine, and passes out of the body. Thus, your body loses its main source of fuel.

SYMPTOMS OF DIABETES

People with diabetes might not have symptoms. When they do, the most common symptoms are

○ excessive thirst
○ excessive hunger
○ excessive urination
○ unintended weight loss
○ tingling or numbness in feet or hands
○ sores that are slow to heal
○ dry, itchy skin

DIABETES IS PREVENTABLE

A large body of evidence shows that certain types of diabetes can be prevented or reversed with good nutrition and exercise.

"I would treat individuals with HIV who are on [HIV medicine] as high-risk cardiovascular patients—without a doubt," says Anthony S. Fauci, M.D., director of the National Institute of Allergy and Infectious Diseases. "In other words, I would say to assume that you have a 45-year-old father who died of a myocardial infarction, your cholesterol is very high, and your mother had diabetes—even though it might not be the case. You have to treat yourself like that. You have to be careful with diet. You have to make sure that you don't fuel an engine of risk that you unfortunately have."

STATES OF THE VIRUS: "ON" OR "OFF"

Eating for *controlled* and *uncontrolled* HIV are two very different situations.

UNCONTROLLED HIV

○ moderate-to-high viral load levels
○ low T-cells

CONTROLLED HIV

○ very low viral levels
○ undetectable (less than 40 copies)

Basics of a healthy diet

The USDA food pyramid is a reasonable diet if you adhere to reasonable portion sizes. But who does? At the same time, fast food and the availability of processed foods—cookies, cake, chips, and soda—have merged to make us fat.

Consensus is building among health professionals that an eating style derived from the Mediterranean region may be healthier than the typical American diet. Sometimes called the Mediterranean diet, this eating style has been well studied because of the notably low incidence of chronic diseases and high life expectancy associated with it.

• • •

TEN PRINCIPLES OF THE MEDITERRANEAN DIET

1. An abundance of food from plant sources, including fruits and vegetables, potatoes, breads and grains, beans, nuts, and seeds
2. Emphasis on a variety of minimally processed and, wherever possible, seasonally fresh and locally grown foods (which often maxi-

mizes the health-promoting micronutrient and antioxidant content
of these foods)

3. Olive oil as the principal fat, replacing other fats and oils (including
   butter and margarine)

4. Total fat ranging from less than 25 percent to over 35 percent of
   energy, with saturated fat no more than 7 to 8 percent of calories

5. Daily consumption of low-to-moderate amounts of cheese and yogurt
   (low-fat and nonfat versions may be preferable)

6. Weekly consumption of low-to-moderate amounts of fish and poultry (recent research suggests that fish should be somewhat favored
   over poultry), from zero to four eggs per week (including those used
   in cooking and baking)

7. Fresh fruit as the typical daily dessert; sweets with a significant
   amount of sugar (often as honey) and saturated fat consumed no
   more than a few times per week

8. Red meat a few times per month (recent research suggests that if red
   meat is eaten, its consumption should be limited to a maximum of 12
   to 16 ounces per month; where the flavor is acceptable, lean versions
   may be preferable)

9. Regular physical activity at a level that promotes a healthy weight, fitness, and well-being

10. Moderate consumption of wine, normally with meals; about one to
    two glasses per day for men and one glass per day for women (wine
    should be considered optional and avoided when consumption would
    put the individual or others at risk)

In a similar way, the American Cancer Society has developed guidelines
for nutrition and cancer prevention. The key principles of this diet include
the following:

○ Choose most of the foods you eat from plant sources.
○ Limit your intake of high-fat foods, particularly from animal sources.
○ Be physically active. Achieve and maintain a healthy weight.

If you do nothing else, do this:

○ Eat more fruits and vegetables every day

Vitamins and supplements are not fruits and vegetables

People who don't like vegetables may try to get by with vitamins. This isn't necessarily a bad idea; it's just not a good one. Studies show that 75 percent of people with HIV use some form of alternative medicine including megavitamins and supplements. But studies done of the general population are also beginning to show that the health benefits of a nutritious diet are not explained by vitamins and supplements alone.

The missing link may be certain substances—besides vitamins and minerals—found only in plants. One name for these substances is phytochemicals, which represent thousands of different components in plant foods.

Phytochemicals are not considered "essential" nutrients. But eating an abundance of phytochemicals from various fruits and vegetables has been associated with the prevention and/or treatment of at least four of the leading causes of death in the United States—cancer, heart disease, diabetes, and high blood pressure.

The specific phytochemical content of different fruits and vegetables tends to vary by color, and each has unique functions. Some phytochemicals act as antioxidants, some protect and regenerate essential nutrients, and others work to deactivate cancer-causing substances.

The top ten food groups that provide the most vitamins, minerals, and phytochemicals include

- Red, yellow, and orange fruits
- Red, yellow, and orange vegetables
- Cruciferous and leafy green vegetables
- Mushrooms
- Sea vegetables
- Garlic and similar plants
- Whole grains
- Beans and other legumes
- Soy and soy products
- Nuts and seeds

Diet, Exercise, and HIV: A Case Study

RESEARCHERS AT Tufts University reported the results of a forty-four-year-old man who was assigned to an intensive diet and exercise regimen for four months. The man had been taking HIV treatment for two-and-a-half-years.

THE PROBLEM:

- ○ gained thirty pounds
- ○ experienced "lipodystrophy," an abnormal body fat condition
- ○ lost body fat in limbs, but gained it in chest and waistline

THE DIET

- ○ consumed at least 25 grams of dietary fiber daily
- ○ 15 percent of total caloric intake from protein
- ○ 30 percent from fat
- ○ 55 percent from carbs

THE EXERCISE

- ○ cardio plus strength training
- ○ 75-minute workout sessions three times a week

THE RESULTS

- ○ lost fourteen pounds
- ○ lowered cholesterol levels
- ○ 28 percent decrease in body fat
- ○ 52 percent decrease in intra-abdominal fat (fat around the internal organs)
- ○ maintained improvements after one year on the regimen

THE LESSON FOR PEOPLE WITH HIV

Researchers concluded that lifestyle solutions—not just pharmaceuticals—can be a powerful treatment for lipodystrophy and many other conditions.

Exercise is good for your heart and head, not your T-cells

It's not true that exercise helps fight HIV. Research has consistently shown that exercise has no effect on T-cells or viral load. End of story.

One caveat: More and more metabolic conditions are being reported among people with HIV. It's not yet clear if these conditions stem from a damaged immune system, the virus itself, or HIV medicine. Some researchers suggest it's a complicated mix of them all.

The conditions include

- ○ fat redistribution (lipodystrophy)
- ○ loss of fat in the extremities (lipoatrophy)
- ○ excess of fat around the internal organs (severe visceral adiposity)
- ○ high cholesterol and triglycerides (lipid abnormalities)
- ○ insulin abnormalities (hyperinsulinemia)
- ○ unusually high blood sugar (hyperglycemia)
- ○ weak bones (osteopenia)

Whatever the true cause, all of these conditions are becoming more common in the HIV population. It puts people with HIV at a higher risk for diabetes, pancreatitis, bone disorders, and heart disease. Exercise is proving to do more than "not hurt." It may actually help. Research is showing that exercise reduces and sometimes eliminates—and may even prevent—these conditions. After all, who wants to survive HIV only to have a heart attack later in life?

Exercise also helps your mind. Research has shown it helps people with HIV cope better with the stresses of life. One study showed that people who were "regular exercisers" had less anxiety and depression after receiving an HIV-positive diagnosis. The researchers concluded that "exercise appeared to provide a 'buffer' to the psychological stress" of living with the virus.

Cope better, and you'll make better health decisions over the long haul. Make better decisions over the long haul, and you'll spin the odds of good fortune in your favor.

• • •

"Inner" fat is worse than garden-variety fat

The most dangerous kind of fat is not what hangs over your belt. The danger lies deep within the belly, behind the stomach muscles. It's called intra-abdominal fat, and as it grows, it wraps around your internal organs and can strangle them. Sometimes, this fat infiltrates your liver.

Inner fat makes people look like the shape of an apple versus the shape of a pear. Among the general population, this particular distribution of fat is more common among older people. People with HIV are more prone to this inner fat for reasons related to the severity of immune depletion and length of time on HIV medicine. Either way, pinching an inch can't tell you how much inner fat lurks on the inside.

Some of the signs of excessive intra-abdominal fat are:

- Heart disease
- High blood pressure
- Stroke
- Type 2 diabetes
- Certain forms of cancer, including uterine, breast, and colon

Exercise shrinks inner fat

"Exercise is amazing," says Anthony S. Fauci, M.D., "Exercise does so many good things for you. It keeps your blood pressure down. It keeps your resting heart rate down. It gives you a level of endorphins that just makes you feel better generally."

Besides making you feel better, moderate exercise can reduce intra-abdominal fat. Researchers at Tufts University studied HIV-positive people, some of whom were taking HIV medicine, while others were not. The researchers found that exercise increased physical functioning, led to weight loss, decreased stomach girth, and reduced fatigue. However, there was no difference in T-cells or virus levels between groups.

A related study found body composition, bone density, and lipid, insulin, and glucose levels all appeared to improve with exercise. The researchers are finding a few guidelines to combat intra-abdominal fat. They include:

- moderate-intensity cardio workout
- resistance training (weight lifting)
- eating well to achieve a healthy weight

Cardio exercise makes your heart beat faster

When you exercise, your heart beats faster to meet the demand for more blood and oxygen by the muscles of the body. The more intense the activity, the faster your heart will beat. Therefore, monitoring your heart rate during exercise can be an excellent way to monitor exercise intensity. According to the American Council on Exercise, the target is to work your heart to about 50 to 80 percent of its capacity.

Maximal Heart Rate: This number is related to your age. As we grow older, our hearts start to beat a little more slowly. To estimate your maximal heart rate, simply subtract your age from the number 220.

Target Heart-Rate Zone: This is the number of beats per minute at which your heart should be beating during cardio exercise.

CALCULATING A CARDIO PLAN

Bob is thirty-six years old and he wants to find his target heart rate.

Step 1

220 minus 36 is 184. This number, 184, is Bob's maximal heart rate.

Step 2

To find Bob's 50 percent heart rate, divide by two. For Bob, that's 92. The number 92 is the minimum number of beats per minute he needs to earn cardio benefits.

Step 3

To find Bob's 80 percent heart rate, use the chart below.

Age:	20	30	40	50	60	70
50%	100	95	90	85	80	75
80%	160	152	144	136	128	120

Now, calculate your target heart rate. However, don't forget the target heart-rate zone is just an estimate. If when you exercise, it feels too hard, it probably is too hard. The time you should keep your heart beating in the target zone depends on many factors.

If you're keeping a health journal, you'll want to write down your target zone and track over time how often you reach the zone.

New physical activity targets included among the National Academy of Sciences Institute of Medicine guidelines say that people should get sixty minutes daily of moderate exercise, such as walking at four miles per hour. The amount recommended by the U.S. Health and Human Services is thirty minutes of moderate exercise each day. The message: exercise between thirty and sixty minutes every day.

HERE ARE A FEW EXAMPLES OF A CARDIO WORKOUT:
- playing volleyball for 45 minutes
- walking 1¾ miles in 35 minutes (20 min/mile)
- bicycling 5 miles in 30 minutes
- dancing fast (social) for 30 minutes
- walking 2 miles in 30 minutes (15 min/mile)
- swimming laps for 20 minutes
- basketball (playing a game) for 15-20 minutes
- bicycling 4 miles in 15 minutes
- running 1½ miles in 15 minutes (10 min/mile)
- shoveling snow for 15 minutes

Strength training builds muscle, tendons, and ligaments

Even if vanity drives you to resistance training, that's fine. Think about it: The vanity benefits come from looking healthy. More resistance training can help you look healthy and be healthy. The benefits won't only be in terms of muscle. Your bones will benefit, too. Your bones will line up better because of stronger connective tissue, called tendons and ligaments. With better tendons and ligaments, you're less prone to injury.

IN A SENTENCE:

> A *nutritious diet with more fruits and vegetables and regular cardio and strength training are more important when you have HIV.*

Key Elements of Strength Training

○ Vary your exercises to work all the major muscle groups. Neglecting certain groups can lead to strength imbalances and postural difficulties.

○ One set of 8–12 repetitions, working the muscle to the point of fatigue, is usually sufficient.

○ Breathe normally throughout the exercise.

○ Lower the resistance with a slow, controlled cadence throughout the full range of motion.

○ Lifting the weight to a count of two and lowering it to a count of three or four is effective.

○ When you are able to perform 12 repetitions of an exercise correctly (without cheating), increase the amount of resistance by 5 to 10 percent to continue safe progress.

○ Aim to exercise each muscle group at least two times per week, with a minimum of two days of rest between workouts.

○ Training more frequently or adding more sets may lead to slightly greater gains, but the small added benefit may not be worth the extra time and effort (not to mention the added risk of injury).

○ Use machines and free weights to provide exercise variety, which is important for both psychological and physiological reasons. Variety not only reduces boredom, but also provides subtle exercise differences that will enhance progress.

American Council on Exercise

HALF-YEAR MILESTONE

You are now halfway through your first year with HIV.

○ YOU KNOW THAT ONLY CERTAIN SEXUAL BEHAVIORS CAN TRANSMIT HIV, AND THAT COMMON SEXUALLY TRANSMITTED DISEASES, SUCH AS HERPES AND HPV, CAN IMPACT YOUR HEALTH IN THE LONG TERM.

○ YOU UNDERSTAND THAT ANXIETY, DEPRESSION, AND THOUGHTS OF SUICIDE ARE COMMON AND NORMAL AND OPTIONS ARE AVAILABLE TO YOU FOR TREATING THESE CONDITIONS.

○ YOU'RE AWARE THAT SUBSTANCE ABUSE, ADDICTION, AND COMPULSIVE BEHAVIOR START WITH YOUR GENES, AND TREATING THESE CONDITIONS CAN IMPROVE YOUR ODDS FOR SUCCESSFUL HIV TREATMENT DOWN THE ROAD.

○ YOU KNOW THAT A NUTRITIOUS DIET WITH MORE FRUITS AND VEGETABLES AND REGULAR CARDIO AND STRENGTH TRAINING ARE IMPORTANT WHEN YOU HAVE HIV.

How to Get the Health Care You Need

THERE MAY come a time when you need medical advice. You might only need simple suggestions on health insurance. Perhaps you need some guidance on accessing Social Security benefits. Maybe you need to see a doctor right away. If you find yourself in a bad spot and you want face-to-face counsel by someone who knows the ropes of living with HIV, your best bet is to contact an AIDS service organization.

AIDS organizations can be lifesavers. These organizations specialize in providing services to people with HIV. One of the greatest services they offer is tried-and-true experience in helping people get access to health care. All the new HIV drugs don't matter much if you can't get them or can't afford to see a doctor.

A recent survey of people with HIV found that 72 percent had incomes of less than $25,000. Only 32 percent had private health insurance and about 20 percent had no health insurance at all. For many people with HIV, becoming affiliated with a local service organization can be the gateway to getting medicine.

"Everybody has to realize if you go into a service organization, it's incredibly bureaucratic," says Jelka Jonker, a counselor at AIDS Project Los Angeles. She explains the reason for the bureaucracy stems from the funds these organizations get from state and federal agencies. These organizations must fulfill certain requirements to prove to their funders that they are, indeed, providing services to the people who need them most.

"It can be frustrating when you first start out," says Jonker, "but it's not impossible. Once you're in the system, however, you have access to a lot of critical things. It's important to know that from the beginning."

Tim L. offers some advice for initially cracking the AIDS service organization system. "Have patience," he says. "You have to go to each organization to get a specific service. You can't expect one organization to have everything. You can't go in there and demand things. You have to be patient. If you sit there and be patient, you get the things you need quicker. If they say they're busy, say 'I don't mind, I'll just sit here and wait.' And you know what? They will get you in."

Cracking the HIV system may take some time, but there is a payoff. There's plenty of experience and knowledge to be found in these organizations. So if you find yourself with questions or concerns about getting good health care—or keeping the health care you have—know that help is out there should you need it.

Service organizations can help with health insurance

There are two types of health insurance: group plans and individual plans. A group health plan is health insurance usually offered by an employer or by a union. Sometimes, these plans allow you to insure dependents as well. An individual plan is insurance sold by HMOs or other issuers to individuals. Remember, although health coverage might be offered through an association, a college, or a group of self-employed individuals, it's probably still considered an "individual" health plan.

Like it or not, an HIV diagnosis makes you a "substandard risk," which means you're an expensive person to keep around. Insurance companies don't like paying for your medical expenses. In fact, some insurance companies will use every trick in the book to drop your coverage.

For group plans, some insurance companies pass these extra expenses on to your employer, which can sometimes be a strike against you since you cost more to insure than the average employee. For individual plans, most insurance companies won't even offer you coverage, and if they do, it will be extremely expensive.

A recent report on the availability of coverage for people with "less than perfect health" showed that HIV-positive people were routinely denied individual coverage. The researchers studied six hypothetical applicants—each with a different medical problem—and all the applicants were given the opportunity to apply for coverage, except the one with HIV.

So if you have health insurance currently, it's a wise idea to keep the plan for as long as possible. One way to do this is by knowing about the Health Insurance Portability and Accountability Act of 1996, known as HIPAA. This relatively new law may:

- increase your ability to get health coverage for yourself and your dependents if you start a new job
- lower your chance of losing existing health care coverage, whether you have the coverage through a job, or through individual health insurance
- help you maintain continuous health coverage for yourself and your dependents when you change jobs
- help you buy health insurance coverage on your own if you lose coverage under an employer's group health plan and have no other health coverage available

Among its specific protections, HIPAA:

- limits the use of "pre-existing condition" exclusions
- prohibits group plans from discriminating by denying you coverage or charging you extra for coverage based on your—or your family's—past or present poor health
- guarantees certain small employers, and certain individuals who lose job-related coverage, the right to purchase health insurance
- guarantees, in most cases, that employers or individuals who purchase health insurance can renew the coverage regardless of any health conditions of individuals covered under the insurance policy

In short, HIPAA may lower your chance of losing existing coverage, ease your ability to switch health plans and/or help you buy coverage on your own if you lose your employer's plan and have no other coverage available. However, HIPAA does not require employers to offer or pay for health coverage. It's no guarantee of health coverage for all workers and it does not eliminate all preexisting condition exclusions. Also remember that you need at least 18 months of previous health insurance coverage—without a significant break in coverage—to take advantage of HIPAA protections.

COBRA *may help when you change jobs*

One federal law that may help you make the most of HIPAA protections is the Consolidated Omnibus Budget Reconciliation Act of 1985 (COBRA). COBRA allows you to keep your health insurance for up to thirty-six months if you leave your job. However, you'll need to pay extra for it. If you worked for a small company with less than twenty employees, your employer does not have to offer COBRA.

If you're between jobs, COBRA can help you avoid a significant break in coverage. That, in turn, may allow you to shorten or eliminate a preexisting condition clause under a new plan offered by a new employer. But remember, COBRA can be very tricky and subject to cumbersome rules and regulations. For example, if you miss just one payment, you can lose COBRA coverage.

If you're concerned about health insurance, ask a specialist

The rules and regulations involved with health insurance, HIPAA, and COBRA are extremely complicated. There's fine print everywhere. Generally, AIDS service organizations can provide you with help in navigating the shark-infested health-insurance waters. As a first step, you can contact the Centers for Medicare & Medicaid Services at (877) 267-2323 or visit their Web site at http://cms.hhs.gov.

The Medical Information Bureau is watching you

The Medical Information Bureau (MIB) is a little like a credit reporting company, but instead of tracking your credit, the MIB tracks your health. If you have ever applied as an individual for life, health, or disability insurance, your name probably is listed with MIB. This company provides details on more than 15 million Americans and Canadians to about 750 insurance companies. MIB claims that the service it provides to insurance companies helps to fight fraud on the part of consumers applying for health coverage.

As with credit reporting agencies, most of the information stays on record with MIB for seven years. Although you are supposed to be notified when someone is checking MIB's database for information about you, it doesn't always happen. For nine dollars, you can request a copy of your

MIB file by logging onto the Medical Information Bureau's Web site at http://www.mib.com.

A word of advice: If you have HIV, think very carefully about applying for health or life insurance. Once MIB has a record of you being denied for insurance, you're considered a substandard risk. This means you could have a rough time finding health, life, or disability insurance in the future.

You can get good health insurance, but it takes persistence

If you do get dinged for having HIV, don't despair. There are high-risk insurance programs designed just for people who can't get health insurance because of serious or expensive medical conditions. These programs are exactly like commercial health insurance in that they charge premiums, copayments, and deductibles for a defined benefits package.

Although the premiums can be a little higher than regular insurance plans, the coverage is usually excellent and surprisingly affordable. For many years, I was covered by a high-risk insurance plan in Illinois. To qualify, I had to prove that I was denied coverage—but that was the easy part.

There's paperwork and details, and a lot of waiting around for forms in the mail. But in the end, I found the coverage to be on par with—or better than—most individual or group insurance plans. If you can't get health insurance any other way, these programs are definitely the way to go. A word of advice: Many of these state-sponsored programs have long waiting periods for enrollment, so start the process early—even if it's just calling for information. You can start the process by calling your state's AIDS hotline (see Resources section) and asking for the telephone number for your state's program.

Programs are available to help you get HIV-related drugs

ADAP (pronounced "ay-dap") is how most people refer to the AIDS Drug Assistance Programs. The programs provide HIV and AIDS-related prescription drugs to people living in the United States and Puerto Rico who don't have health insurance or who have inadequate health insurance. The program started in 1987 and was dramatically expanded during the 1990s. Every year, Congress allots a certain amount of money to individual states to spend on these programs and this funding can vary from year to year, depending on national fiscal and political trends.

When Congress gives the money to the states, it mandates that the money be spent to "provide therapeutics to treat HIV disease or prevent the serious deterioration of health arising from HIV diseases in eligible individuals, including measures for the prevention and treatment of opportunistic infections."

From there, individual states determine the criteria that a person must meet in order to qualify for the program in that state. For example, you might qualify for New York's program but not for the program in Texas. The states also decide which specific drugs they will offer. So you might have access to a certain drug if you live in California, but not if you live Florida. Both the criteria that a person must meet to be eligible and the drugs offered by the programs can vary from year to year.

Examples of Eligibility in ADAP

EVERY YEAR the eligibility for ADAP changes. Two examples of the criteria to qualify for ADAP are listed below to give you a sense the requirements.

NORTH CAROLINA
○ Your income must be at or below 125 percent of the current federal poverty level (in 2007, the poverty level was $10,210, so your income must be at or below $12,762)
○ You must be HIV-positive
○ You must be a resident of North Carolina
○ You must have no private health insurance or Medicaid
○ A limited number of people can be in the program, so there is a waiting list

MICHIGAN
○ Your income must be at or below 450 percent of the current federal poverty level (so your income must be at or below $45,945)
○ You must be HIV-positive
○ You must be a resident of Michigan
○ You must first apply for Medicaid and have been recently denied
○ You cannot be eligible for Veteran's benefits

Getting started: Use the Resources section in this book to find your state's AIDS hotline. The hotline will provide you with the specific details of your state's ADAP program.

Joining a clinical trial is one way to get medical care

Clinical trials are carefully designed studies that examine the safety and effectiveness of experimental treatments. Clinical trials test the effectiveness of new drugs, test standard medications in different dosages, and compare different combinations of medications to see which ones are most effective. Some clinical trials simply observe your behavior without adding or changing medications

Some trials investigate and treat HIV in patients, while others treat complications and co-infections that may accompany HIV, such as opportunistic infections, hepatitis C, hepatitis B, and tuberculosis (TB). But like anything else, there are pros and cons to be weighed.

ADVANTAGES OF JOINING A CLINICAL TRIAL
○ benefits from the new treatment
○ free laboratory tests and results
○ access to treatments not available to the public
○ free supplies of standard or new drugs
○ regular medical examinations
○ satisfaction from improving the care of others with HIV

DISADVANTAGES OF JOINING A CLINICAL TRIAL
○ taking new drugs that have no benefit or have negative long-term consequences
○ not knowing whether you are receiving the actual therapeutic drug or a placebo
○ more frequent visits for care than would otherwise be necessary
○ being restricted from using other treatments or participating in other studies because of requirements of the clinical trial

For information about participating in clinical trials or trial availability throughout the US, call the AIDS Treatment Information Service (ATIS) at (800) 874-2572 or call a local AIDS service organization.

Social Security can be a lifeline for people with HIV

Social Security benefits come in several forms. Three that are especially important are Medicaid, Social Security Disability Insurance (SSDI), and Supplemental Security Income (SSI).

MEDICAID

Medicaid is a health insurance program offered by the federal government. Its purpose is to help people with especially low incomes, such as children, pregnant women, the elderly, and people with special disabilities such as AIDS. Medicaid will pay for a variety of medical services, including visits to the hospital, visits to the doctor, blood tests, home health care, and family planning.

In most cases, childless adults living with HIV qualify for Medicaid only after they qualify for Supplemental Security Income (SSI). To be eligible for SSI, you must be disabled. HIV-positive people without symptoms don't automatically qualify for Medicaid until they have full-blown AIDS. However, some states have a special arrangement with the federal government, allowing these states to extend Medicaid benefits to nondisabled people living with HIV.

SOCIAL SECURITY DISABILITY INSURANCE (SSDI)

Most people qualify for Social Security disability by working, paying Social Security taxes, and in turn, earning "credits" toward eventual benefits. The dollar amount of your benefit depends on how much you earned in the past. Generally, higher earnings mean higher benefits. You can—and should—keep track of your earning history. If you find a discrepancy, have it corrected sooner rather than later.

SUPPLEMENTAL SECURITY INCOME (SSI)

SSI is a program that pays monthly benefits to people with low incomes and limited assets who are sixty-five or older, blind, or disabled. SSI supplements your income up to a certain level. The level varies from one state to another.

There are a lot of complicated rules about what specifically counts as income, so this is one area where an AIDS service organization can really come in handy. If you work, there are even more rules. People on SSI should have limited assets. Generally, your assets should be under $2,000, or for couples, your assets should be under $3,000. But your home, personal belongings, and car don't count (unless it's an expensive one).

Defining "disability" can be tricky

Disability under Social Security is based on your inability to work. You're considered disabled if you can't do the work you did before and can't adjust to other work because of your medical condition. If you have HIV and have

How Does Social Security Evaluate Your Disability?

SOCIAL SECURITY works with an agency in each state, usually called a Disability Determination Service, to evaluate disability claims. It's a step-by-step process involving five questions:

Step 1—*Are you working?*
If you are working *and* your earnings average more than $700 a month, you're generally not considered disabled.

Step 2—*Is your condition "severe"?*
Your condition must interfere with basic work-related activities.

Step 3—*Is your condition found in a list of "disabling impairments"?*
Social Security maintains a list of "impairments" that are so severe they automatically mean you're disabled. If your condition isn't on the list, your condition must be equal in severity to an impairment that is on the list. For women and children with HIV, the list includes some unique impairments. Some of the HIV-related conditions are:

○ Pulmonary tuberculosis resistant to treatment
○ Kaposi's sarcoma (KS)
○ *Pneumocystis carinii* pneumonia (PCP)
○ Cancer of the cervix
○ Herpes
○ Hodgkin's disease and all lymphomas
○ HIV wasting
○ Syphilis and Neurosyphilis
○ Candidiasis (thrush)

Step 4—*Can you do the work you did previously?*
If your condition is severe—but not of equal severity as the ones on the list—then you must prove that it interferes with your ability to do the work.

Step 5—*Can you do any other type of work?*
Your medical condition, age, education, past work experience, and any transferable skills are considered.

symptoms that severely limit your ability to work—and if you meet the other eligibility factors—the chances are good that you'll qualify for benefits. On the other hand, if you have HIV but no symptoms, it is much harder to qualify for benefits. Social Security officials are becoming stricter with these rules.

Document your impairments

You'll need to document all of your impairments. This may include medical records and blood test results. Remember, you'll need to prove that you have HIV *and* any related conditions. This may include repeated infections; fevers; night sweats; enlarged lymph nodes, liver or spleen; lower energy or general weakness; cough; depression and anxiety; headache; nausea and vomiting; and side effects of your HIV medicine, and how they affect your daily activities.

Not all doctors are aware of all the kinds of information Social Security needs to document your disability. Ask your doctor or other health-care provider to track your symptoms in detail over time and to keep a thorough record of fatigue, depression, forgetfulness, dizziness, and other hard-to-document symptoms.

It's also critical to document how you function day-to-day. This is where your health journal can come in handy. Use your health journal to jot down brief notes about how you feel on each day. Record anything that shows that you couldn't do your regular activities. Be specific. Don't forget to include any psychological problems or how it's affected your job, if you are working.

Bring every detail and document when you apply for benefits

You can apply for Social Security and SSI disability benefits by calling or visiting any Social Security office. In addition, AIDS service organizations usually have on hand most of the documents you need to get the paperwork going. Before making the trip to a Social Security office or an AIDS service organization, be sure to bring your

- Social Security number
- birth certificate
- copy of most recent W-2 form (tax return if you're self-employed)
- documentation of how your condition affects your daily activities

    O   names and addresses of previous doctors and clinics
    O   summary of work history
    O   blood-test results or lab work

If you're signing up for SSI, you'll need to provide records that show that your income and assets are below the SSI limits. This usually includes bank statements, rental receipts, or car registration.

Social Security officials often have special arrangements with AIDS service organizations to streamline the claims process. In some emergency situations, you might qualify for up to six months of benefits before a final decision on your claim. For more information, call Social Security directly at (800) 772-1213 or call a local AIDS service organization listed in the Resource Guide in the back of this book.

IN A SENTENCE:

> AIDS organizations help you with health-care issues, such as getting and keeping health insurance, programs for prescription drugs, and social security.

learning

How to Spot HIV Discrimination

LOUIS HOLIDAY wanted to become a police officer for the city of Chattanooga, Tennessee. He was qualified: He passed a written exam and a physical agility test, consisting of running, jumping hurdles, treading an obstacle course, and carrying heavy weights. In fact, a conditional offer of employment was extended to Holiday, if he passed a psychological and physical examination.

During the physical exam, Holiday informed the doctor he was HIV-positive, even though the city doesn't normally test applicants for HIV, or have a policy that requires applicants to test negative for the virus. Subsequently, Holiday was informed that the city's conditional offer of employment was withdrawn because he had not passed the physical examination.

When Holiday asked why, the city responded that it didn't want to "put other employees and the public at risk by hiring you." The city claimed that Holiday's HIV status posed a health and safety threat to others because of the possibility of blood-to-blood contact during police work. After some time, however, the city recanted because there was no evidence that this was a reasonable assumption. Instead, the city claimed Holiday's HIV played absolutely no role in its decision to withdraw the employment offer.

Holiday suspected otherwise. He took the matter to court on the premise that his rights under the law had been violated by refusing to hire him solely because of his HIV status. The court agreed, saying that Holiday "was entitled to be evaluated based on his actual abilities and relevant medical evidence, and to be protected from discrimination founded on fear, ignorance, and misconceptions."

"This ruling makes it clear that medically related employment decisions, whether they are about HIV or any other disability, must be based on facts about the individual, not based solely on opinion," said Matthew Coles, director of the American Civil Liberties Union's AIDS Project. For employers, the message is clear: You cannot discriminate against employees or job applicants just because they have HIV.

If you have HIV, you have some protections under the law. Even people who don't have the virus are discriminated against because they're regarded as having HIV. They're protected too.

Our founding fathers guaranteed us a few things

First, understand that you've been granted a basic level of "guarantees" by the federal government. These guarantees are based on the concept that all men are created equal and that the creator of all men—some call this God—has given you the right to life, liberty, and the pursuit of happiness. Of course, how the United States federal government interprets these minimum guarantees changes over time.

At one time in the United States, you could be enslaved because you were black. At another time in history, you could be jailed because you were Japanese. More recently, you could be denied a job because you were a woman.

In 1990, people with HIV got a certain set of guarantees from the federal government. These came in the form of the Americans with Disabilities Act, more commonly known as the ADA. If you have HIV, you're legally considered "disabled." It doesn't mean you can't walk or need a wheelchair, it only means that you have a few more physical challenges than the average American.

Before the ADA, the consensus was that people with disabilities should be institutionalized, that they were a lower class and should be kept out of sight. The disability rights movement is similar to the civil rights movements before it. Before 1990, it had been assumed that hardships of people with disabilities, such as unemployment and lack of health care, were due to the disability itself, and not the way society reacted to the disability.

After 1990, excluding and segregating people with disabilities was viewed as discrimination.

Basically, if you have HIV and you're a citizen of the United States, you're considered disabled. If you're disabled and a citizen of the United States, you're legally protected from discrimination. Now, it doesn't mean that it can't happen, it only means that you can do something about it.

The first step is recognizing discrimination

Discrimination happens all the time to people with HIV. It even happens to people who are HIV-negative because it's assumed that they have the virus. How do you spot discrimination? Well, the definition changes depending on time and location.

If you live in Massachusetts in 2007, you're protected from HIV discrimination exceptionally well. The problem is that laws are different in each state. Most laws attempt to stop discrimination, but people don't always agree on how to enforce these laws.

Checklist for proving discrimination

IN A court of law, you usually have to prove a few things before you can legally claim you've been discriminated against. Here are a few of the basic things you must prove:

- **Action and Inaction:** you have to prove that someone *did* something or *did not do* something that causes you harm or injury.
- **Harm and Injury:** you have to prove that something bad—on a physical level—has happened to you, or you were denied the opportunity to get something good.
- **Disparate or Unequal Treatment:** You were treated differently or worse than others because you have HIV.
- **Disparate or Unequal Impact:** This basically means that sometimes certain rules are unfair—even when the rules attempt to be fair.
- **Separate Treatment:** This happens when you're treated differently for irrational reasons.

Laws are like tools: They only help if you use them. Sometimes, just sharing your understanding of the law with the right people—at the right time—can solve your problems, and save everyone time, money, and grief. Other times, you may need to take a stand or make people obey the law.

Louis Holiday went to court because he wanted to make the point that people with disabilities ought to be judged on the basis of their abilities; that they should not be judged nor discriminated against based on unfounded fear, prejudice, ignorance, or mythologies; people ought to be judged on the relevant medical evidence and the abilities they have. The court agreed.

The ADA spells out your protections

The ADA gives civil rights protections to people with HIV in a similar way to those provided to people with issues of race, color, sex, national origin, age, and religion. It guarantees equal opportunity for people with disabilities in public accommodations, employment, transportation, and state and local government services. If you have HIV, you're protected by the law. Persons who are discriminated against because they are regarded as being HIV-positive are also protected.

The ADA makes rules for dos and don'ts in employment situations

The ADA prohibits discrimination by all private employers with fifteen or more employees. In addition, the ADA prohibits all public entities, regardless of the size of their workforce, from discriminating in employment against qualified individuals with disabilities.

The ADA prohibits discrimination in all employment practices. This includes not only hiring and firing, but job application procedures (including the job interview), job assignment, training, and promotions. It also includes wages, benefits (including health insurance), leave, and all other employment-related activities.

IN REAL LIFE:

Examples of *employment discrimination* against people with HIV include:

○ An automobile manufacturing company had a blanket policy of refusing to hire anyone infected with HIV.
○ An airline extended an offer to a job applicant and then rescinded the offer when, after the applicant took an HIV test as part of the airline's required medical examination, the applicant tested positive.

- A restaurant fired a waitress after learning that the waitress had HIV.
- A university fired a physical education instructor after learning that the instructor's boyfriend had HIV.
- A company contracted with an insurance company that had a cap on health insurance benefits provided to employees for HIV complications, but not on other health insurance benefits.

"Reasonable accommodation" can be a slight moderation

A "reasonable accommodation" is any modification or adjustment to a job, the job application process, or the work environment that will enable a qualified applicant or employee with a disability to perform the essential functions of the job, participate in the application process, or enjoy the benefits and privileges of employment.

Examples include: making existing facilities readily accessible to and usable by employees with disabilities; restructuring a job; modifying work schedules; acquiring or modifying equipment; and reassigning a current employee to a vacant position for which the individual is qualified.

IN REAL LIFE:

Examples of *reasonable accommodation* for people with HIV include:

- An HIV-positive accountant required two hours off, bimonthly, for visits to his doctor. He was permitted to take longer lunch breaks and to make up the time by working later on those days.
- An HIV-positive computer programmer suffered bouts of nausea caused by his medication. His employer allowed him to work at home on those days that he found it too difficult to come into the office. His employer provided him with the equipment (computer, modem, fax machine, etc.) necessary for him to work at home.

An employer is not required to make an accommodation if it would impose an undue hardship on the operation of the business. An undue hardship is an action that requires "significant difficulty or expense" in relation to the size of the employer, the resources available, and the nature of the operation. Determination as to whether a particular accommodation poses an undue hardship must be made on a case-by-case basis.

• • •

Customer or coworker attitudes are not relevant. The potential loss of customers or coworkers because an employee has HIV does not constitute an undue hardship. An employer is not required to provide an employee's first choice of accommodation. The employer is required to provide an effective accommodation that meets the individual's needs.

An employer is only required to accommodate a "known" disability of a qualified applicant or employee. Thus, it is the employee's responsibility to tell the employer that he or she needs a reasonable accommodation. If the employee doesn't want to disclose HIV status, it may be sufficient for the employee to say that he or she has an illness or disability covered by the ADA, that the illness or disability causes certain problems with work, and that the employee wants a reasonable accommodation. However, an employer can require medical documentation of the employee's disability and the limitations resulting from that disability.

Sometimes employers are concerned about the future

Employers cannot choose *not* to hire a qualified person now because they fear the worker will become too ill to work in the future. The hiring decision must be based on how well the individual can perform now. In addition, employers cannot decide to *not* hire qualified people with HIV or AIDS because they are afraid of higher medical insurance costs, workers compensation costs, or absenteeism.

Some employers can consider safety when hiring people with HIV

An employer may consider health and safety when deciding whether to hire an applicant or retain an employee who has HIV only under limited circumstances. The ADA permits employers to establish qualification standards that will exclude individuals who pose a direct threat—i.e., a significant risk of substantial harm—to the health or safety of the individual or of others, if that risk cannot be eliminated or reduced below the level of a "direct threat" by reasonable accommodation.

However, an employer may not simply assume that a threat exists; the employer must establish through objective, medically supportable methods that there is a significant risk that substantial harm could occur in the workplace. By requiring employers to make individualized judgments based on reliable medical or other objective evidence—rather than on generalizations, ignorance, fear, patronizing attitudes, or stereotypes.

The ADA recognizes the need to balance the interests of people with disabilities against the legitimate interests of employers in maintaining a safe workplace. Transmission of HIV will rarely be a legitimate "direct threat" issue.

It is medically established that HIV can only be transmitted by sexual contact with an infected individual, exposure to infected blood or blood products, or perinatally from infected mother to infant during pregnancy, birth, or breastfeeding. HIV cannot be transmitted by casual contact. Thus, there is little possibility that HIV could ever be transmitted in the workplace.

In Real Life:

Examples of *assumed threat* and HIV include:

- A superintendent may believe that there is a risk of employing an individual with HIV as a schoolteacher. However, there is little or no likelihood of a direct exchange of body fluids between the teacher and her students, and thus, employing this person would not pose a direct threat.
- A restaurant owner may believe that there is a risk of employing an individual with HIV as a cook, waiter or waitress, or dishwasher, because the employee might transmit the disease through the handling of food. However, HIV and AIDS are specifically not included on the Centers for Disease Control and Prevention list of infectious and communicable diseases that are transmitted through the handling of food. Thus, there is little or no likelihood that employing persons with HIV in food handling positions would pose a risk of transmitting HIV.
- A fire chief may believe that an HIV-positive firefighter may pose a risk to others when performing mouth-to-mouth resuscitation. However, current medical evidence indicates that HIV cannot be transmitted by the exchange of saliva. Thus, there is little or no likelihood that an HIV-infected firefighter would pose a risk to others.

Having HIV can impair your ability to do the job

Having HIV might impair your ability to perform certain functions of a job, thus causing the individual to pose a direct threat to the health or safety of the individual or others.

IN REAL LIFE:
Examples of *direct threat* and HIV include:

○ A worker who operates heavy machinery and who has been suffering from dizzy spells caused by the medication he is taking might pose a direct threat to his or someone else's safety. If no reasonable accommodation is available (e.g., an open position to which the employee could be reassigned), the employer would not violate the ADA by laying off the worker.

○ An airline pilot who is experiencing bouts of dementia would pose a direct threat to the safety of passengers. It would not violate the ADA if the airline prohibited her from flying. As noted above, the direct threat assessment must be an individualized assessment.

Any blanket exclusion—for example, refusing to hire persons with HIV because of the attendant health risks—would probably violate the ADA as a matter of law.

Employers should not ask about HIV

An employer may not ask or require a job applicant to take a medical examination before making a job offer. It cannot make any preoffer inquiry about a disability or the nature or severity of a disability. However, an employer may ask questions about the ability to perform specific job functions.

After a person starts work, a medical examination or inquiry of an employee must be job-related and consistent with business necessity. Employers may conduct employee medical examinations where there is evidence of a job performance or safety problem, when examinations are required by other federal laws, when examinations are necessary to determine current "fitness" to perform a particular job, and/or where voluntary examinations are part of employee health programs.

Employers should keep your HIV status confidential

The ADA requires that medical information be kept confidential. This information must be kept apart from general personnel files as a separate, confidential medical record available only under limited conditions.

Employers shouldn't discriminate with health insurance

The ADA prohibits employers from discriminating on the basis of disability in the provision of health insurance to their employees and/or from entering into contracts with health insurance companies that discriminate on the basis of disability.

Insurance distinctions that are not based on disability, however, and that are applied equally to all insured employees, do not discriminate on the basis of disability and do not violate the ADA.

Thus, for example, blanket preexisting condition clauses that exclude from the coverage of a health insurance plan the treatment of all physical conditions that predate an individual's eligibility for benefits are not distinctions based on disability and do not violate the ADA. A preexisting condition clause that excluded only the treatment of HIV-related conditions is a disability-based distinction and would likely violate the ADA.

If you think you've been discriminated against in employment

If you believe that you've been discriminated against, the first step is to try to educate the employer about what the ADA requires. If the issue isn't resolved satisfactorily, you can file a complaint with the nearest Equal Employment Opportunity Commission office within 180 days of when the discrimination occurred.

This office will investigate the complaint and either act to correct the problem or give the employee a "right to sue" letter. The right-to-sue letter permits the employee to sue the employer directly. The employee may be entitled to the job he or she was denied, back pay, benefits, or other compensatory and punitive damages.

For more information about the ADA's employment requirements, call Equal Employment Opportunity Commission at (800) 669-4000.

ADA prohibits state and local governments from discriminating because of HIV

The ADA applies to all state and local governments, their departments and agencies, and any other instrumentalities or special-purpose districts of state or local governments.

IN REAL LIFE:
Examples of *state or local discrimination* and HIV include:

○ A public school system prohibits an HIV-positive child from attending elementary school.
○ A county hospital refuses to treat persons with HIV.
○ A state-owned nursing home refuses to accept patients with HIV. A
county recreation center refuses admission to a summer-camp
program for a child whose brother has HIV.

If you think that state or city government is discriminating against you or your family

If you believe that you're being discriminated against by a state or local
government, first try to educate officials involved about the ADA's requirements. You may also file a complaint with the Department of Justice.
Complaints must be filed within 180 days of when the discrimination
occurred.

COMPLAINTS SHOULD BE SENT TO:
US Department of Justice
Civil Rights Division
Disability Rights Section
Post Office Box 66738
Washington, D.C. 20035-6738

As a last resort, you can sue the pants off them

You also have the right to bring private ADA lawsuits against state and
local governments to seek relief, compensatory damages, and reasonable
attorney's fees.

ADA Employment questions
(800) 669-4000

ADA Employment documents
(800) 669-3362

FDA Office of AIDS and Special Health Issues
(301) 827-4460

National AIDS Program Office
(202) 690-5560

IN A SENTENCE:

> *Having HIV might result in discrimination, but you have some protections under the law.*

When to Start HIV Medicine

IF THERE'S one person who sees the big picture of HIV medicine, it's Anthony Fauci, M.D. Since 1980, he's been the director of the National Institute of Allergy and Infectious Diseases (NIAID), a U.S. government agency that supports research and sets policy to prevent, diagnose, and treat infectious and immune-related illnesses, including HIV and other sexually transmitted diseases.

"People with HIV need to start thinking not just in terms of the virus, but in the totality of their health," says Dr. Fauci. "Like any other condition, you're treating the *whole* person. The whole person has many other things going on. You're not just treating a virus."

Your own big picture must take into account all the aspects that make up your life and your health. Some aspects of your life may have little to do with medicine. For example, you might be between jobs or concerned about money. You might not have health insurance or access to good medical care. For others, substance-abuse issues may be more urgent these days. In fact, you'll benefit more from HIV medicine if you're not using drugs or alcohol.

Then there are medical aspects that may be unrelated to HIV. You may also have chronic hepatitis C virus (HCV) or chronic hepatitis B virus (HBV). In some cases, the decision to treat HCV or HBV will likely influence your plan to treat HIV. These are all factors that figure into your decision to start—or not start—HIV treatment.

T-cell count tests measure how far HIV disease has progressed

A normal T-cell count is between 500 and 1600, although results can vary a little due to the time of day, fatigue, and stress. Infections and vaccinations can have a large impact on your T-cell counts. It's best to have blood drawn at the same time of day and to not check your T-cells until a couple of weeks after you recover from an infection, or after you get a vaccination.

350 AND HIGHER T-CELLS

If your T-cells are above 350, your risk of progressing to AIDS within three years is relatively low. A T-cell count of 350 or higher generally means that HIV has not progressed very far. Of course, the higher the number, the better. However, when your T-cells are consistently above 350, your immune system is in relatively good shape. You should be able to fight infections fairly well.

When considering HIV medicine, you should know that people with 350 or more T-cells tend to report more long-term side effects. In fact, 40 percent of people with high T-cells switched medications due to side effects and 20 percent discontinued medicine after two years. Since the risk of disease progression is low, you should weigh this fact against potential risks of HIV medicine, how it may affect your quality of life, and how you will respond to future treatments. You should also consider your viral load. For many people with high T-cells, the risks of HIV medicine are greater than the risks of disease progression.

200 TO 350 T-CELLS

If your T-cells are between 200 and 350, your risk of progressing to AIDS within three years is significantly higher. This means that HIV has already progressed somewhat and has done some damage to your immune system. However, this category is the gray zone of HIV medicine. Some serious illnesses, especially tuberculosis and pneumonia, can occur when your T-cells are above 200. When considering HIV treatment, you should know that people generally do worse on medicine when their T-cells are around 200 when compared to people with higher T-cells. Some of these poor responses include:

○ slower increase in T-cells count after starting medicine
○ decreased ability to lower viral load to below the limit of detection
○ increased ability of HIV to become resistant to treatment

If your T-cells are in between 200 and 350, your viral load is far more important in tipping the scales to treat or delay treatment. If your viral load is high, there's a much greater risk for progressing to AIDS.

200 OR LESS T-CELLS

If your T-cells are less than 200, this is not good. Your immune system has been severely damaged by HIV and you may not be able to fight infections. You will need to take special medicine to prevent certain diseases (notably a certain form of pneumonia) and start HIV medicine immediately. Studies have shown that people sometimes do worse on medicine because their T-cells were below 200 when they started it. HIV treatment should not be delayed if your T-cell count is below 200.

Viral load tests measure how fast HIV is progressing

To measure HIV levels in your blood, doctors use viral load tests, which are also called assays. There are several different kinds of viral load tests and they all give results in slightly different ways. All three of the main types of viral tests—PCR, bDNA and NASBA—give your HIV viral load result in terms of *RNA levels* or *copies*. Sometimes, the companies that run the viral load tests provide your doctor with test results that are specific to the type of viral load test. For example, a PCR test result might not be the same as a bDNA result. However, your doctor should translate the results to the standard RNA levels or copies. The three main types of viral load tests are:

○ PCR (HIV RNA reverse transcription-polymerase chain reaction) give results in a range between 400 and 750,000 copies. There's an ultra-sensitive test that gives results between 50 and 75,000 copies.
○ bDNA (branched chain DNA) gives viral load results in a range of between 75 and 500,000 copies.

○ NASBA (nucleic acid sequence-based amplification) gives viral load results between 40 and 10,000,000 copies. There's a special test that gives a range of 50 to 3 million copies.

The best viral load test result is *undetectable*. However, this does not mean that there is no virus in your blood; it just means that there is not enough for the test to find and count. For example, with a PCR test undetectable could mean 399 copies. However, the same result would not be undetectable if an ultra-sensitive test was used.

Know where your T-cells and viral load are heading

T-cells and viral loads are complicated enough, but it's important to remember that a single T-cell count and viral load result is just a snapshot of a moving target. You should consider where your T-cells and viral load are headed in general. Are your T-cells declining quickly? Or are they staying stable over time? In the same way, knowing if your viral load is increasing or decreasing over time helps you get a better picture of your health.

"If a month ago you were at 1,000 [T-cells], then two weeks later you were at 700, and today you're at 400, that's quite different than having 400 a month ago and today you're at 420. In the later case, you're obviously not sloping down," says Dr. Fauci.

T-cells are only half the picture. The other half is your viral load, which is especially important if your T-cells are between 200 and 350. For example, if you had 290 T-cells and a low viral load (less than 20,000 copies), some doctors may want to start you on treatment while others may not. If you had 290 T-cells and a high viral load (greater than 50,000 copies), most doctors would agree that starting medicine is a good decision.

Hit hard, but wait longer

HIV research is constantly changing. Years ago, conventional wisdom held that people with HIV should treat the virus at any stage in the hope that the virus would be eradicated from the body. This strategy was called "hit hard, and hit early." It's based on the idea that patient should take the most potent HIV drugs as early as possible. Studies found this strategy wasn't possible and long-term side effects became more of a problem.

What does your viral load mean?

Less than 50

If your viral load is less than 50 copies, many doctors will report this as "undetectable." This is great news. This means that HIV has basically been stopped in its tracks.

Less than 400

If your viral load is less than 400 copies, this is good news for now. This means that HIV is progressing very slowly. Some doctors may inaccurately report a viral load of less than 400 as "undetectable." Keep in mind that a viral load of less than 400 is not as good as less than 50. Be sure to ask what the lower limit of detection is for the viral load test your doctor performed.

Between 400 and 5,000

If your viral load is in between 400 and 5,000, this is not ideal, but it isn't bad news. A viral load in this range is generally considered on the low end of the scale. It means that HIV is progressing at a slow-to-moderate pace.

Between 5,000 and 30,000

Another gray area of HIV treatment is when a viral load falls between 5,000 and 30,000. This means that HIV is progressing at a moderate pace. On one hand, AIS recommends you begin medicine if your viral load is between 5,000 and 30,000 and you have a T-cell count of less than 500. On the other hand, the U.S. Department of Health and Human Services (DHHS) guidelines say that if you have a viral load below 55,000 and more than 350 T-cells, you don't need to start treatment.

Between 30,000 and 55,000

If your viral load is in the range of 30,000 and 55,000, it means that your HIV is progressing relatively fast. IAS recommends treatment if your viral load is greater than 30,000 regardless of your T-cell count.

Above 55,000

By all measures, a viral load result of greater than 55,000 is considered high and HIV progression is moving very quickly. For example, one study of people with T-cell counts of 201 to 350 and who had a viral load of greater than 55,000 found that the risk of progression to AIDS within three years was about 64 percent. But don't sweat it, HIV medicine is very effective at reducing the viral load.

"Hit hard, but wait longer" is the new mantra for treating HIV. This new strategy is based on a large and growing body of research that shows very little benefit for people who start treatment when their T-cells are above 350. For people with T-cells between 200 and 350, the decision is a judgment call, one that should take the totality of your health into account. Several recent studies have shown that starting therapy when your T-cell counts are between 200 and 350 might mean fewer problems and a lower cost of care because of the fewer complications. If your T-cells are higher than 350, taking treatment may be worse for your health than taking nothing at all.

"When you're dealing with a disease in which the primary issue is cataclysmic—such as life or death due to the virus itself—there's very little wiggle room about what you should do, about whether you should treat or not," says Dr. Fauci. Once the medical community takes control of a disease and longevity is common for most people with the disease, then "secondary issues" begin to rise in importance.

Recent studies have shown that HIV medicine is associated with increases in heart disease and metabolic abnormalities. According to Dr. Fauci, the side effects from HIV medicine that are now emerging are just the tip of the iceberg: "Whenever you have major perturbations from an infection or chronic administration of powerful drugs, it's amazing what you see five, ten, fifteen, and twenty years down the pike."

However, it's important to remember that a potential increase in risk for heart disease does not mean that you will get heart disease. According to Bob Munk, a long-time HIV treatment advocate who has also been HIV-positive for over twenty years, people considering treatment ought to put things in proper perspective. "I see people who are freaked out that the risk of heart disease may go up 1 percent without putting it in context that the risk of HIV disease progression and death has gone down by 80 percent."

A sound approach for dealing with long-term side effects is to be ready for them, says Dr. Fauci. In this way, you're better able to prevent them from happening or reduce the damage if they do happen. "You have to think in terms of the delicate balance between being aggressive enough to suppress the virus and conservative enough not to inappropriately treat a person that doesn't really need to be treated."

Guidelines can help you decide when to treat HIV

Treatment guidelines and strategies have emerged to help patients and doctors better understand the risks of HIV medicine versus the risks of not treating the virus. Physicians, researchers, and consumers in conjunction with the U.S. Department of Health and Human Services (DHHS) developed one set of treatment guidelines. HIV researchers and physicians in conjunction with the International AIDS Society-USA (IAS), a nonprofit physician education organization, created another set of guidelines, which often focus more on areas where there is controversy or insufficient research for definitive approaches to care or treatment.

Taken together, both documents represent the latest thinking about HIV medicine and serve as roadmaps for people with the virus. Both documents are revised regularly—sometimes from year to year—so it's important to keep track of any major changes that might affect your decisions about treatment.

Both documents are available on the Internet. The DHHS document, called the "Guidelines for the Use of Antiretroviral Agents in HIV-Infected Adults and Adolescents" is available at www.aidsinfo.nih.gov. The IAS document, called the "Updated Recommendations for the Use of Antiretroviral Therapy," is available at www.iasusa.org.

The following are tables from both treatment guidelines and they reflect two opinions. Both guidelines can be intimidating for people without medical training. To make things more complicated, the HIV research changes all the time. But the changes are not dramatic from year to year. Rather, the changes are just refinements of tried and true approaches to treating HIV. Within the medical community, there is a consensus about the primary goals of HIV medicine. The goals include:

- preserving your immune system
- lowering your viral load as much as possible for as long as possible
- minimizing side effects from treatment
- reducing sickness and death due to HIV

IAS-USA RECOMMENDATIONS FOR WHEN TO START THERAPY

T-cell count	Viral load (copies)		
	Less than 5,000	5,000–30,000	Greater than 30,000
Less than 350	Recommend treatment	Recommend treatment	Recommend treatment
350 to 500	Consider treatment	Recommend treatment	Recommend treatment
Greater than 500	Defer treatment	Consider treatment	Recommend treatment

DHHS RECOMMENDATIONS FOR WHEN TO START THERAPY

Clinical category	T-cell count	Viral load (copies)	Recommendation
Severe symptoms	Any value	Any value	Treat
No symptoms	Less than 200	Any value	Treat
No symptoms	Between 200–350	Any value	HIV medicine should generally be offered, though controversy exists
No symptoms	Greater than 350	Greater than 55,000	Some experts would recommend medicine, since the three-year risk of developing AIDS in untreated patients is greater than 30 percent; some would defer medicine and monitor T-cells and viral load more frequently
No symptoms	Greater than 350	Less than 55,000	Many experts would defer medicine, since three-year risk of developing AIDS in untreated patients is less than 15 percent

IN A SENTENCE:

Understand where your T-cell counts and viral load are heading so you can make an informed decision about when to start HIV medicine.

learning

Choosing the Best HIV Medicine

ONCE YOU decide to start HIV medicine, the next step is choosing which ones are best for you. For over fifteen years, I've written about HIV medications and I've taken them myself. Today, I'm happily alive. I feel the benefit of medicine each morning when I wake up. But also I feel the side effects. When I put on a pair of jeans, the shape of my body just doesn't feel right. As with every drug, there are pros and cons.

There are four general classes of HIV drugs: nukes, non-nukes, protease inhibitors, and fusion inhibitors. Keep in mind that fusion inhibitors are used as *salvage therapy* if someday your current HIV drugs stop working. The focus of this chapter is on *first-line therapy,* which is a combination of three HIV drugs for people who have *never* taken HIV drugs before. People in this category are called *drug naïve* (this doesn't mean you're not smart, it means your body hasn't been exposed to HIV drugs).

If you're drug naïve, you have the highest chance of success with HIV medicine. You're likely to get the most benefit, with the fewest side effects, over the longest period of time. When it comes to having success with HIV medicine, your first shot is your best shot. Creating a second- or third-line HIV regimen becomes more complicated. Second-line treatment is discussed later in this book. This chapter, however, focuses only on the preferred HIV drugs for first-line treatment.

I say the ideal HIV medicine available these days is Atripla. Do I take Atripla? Well, almost. It's complicated. Atripla is manufactured by two different pharmaceutical companies and although it comes in one pill, it's actually composed of three different drugs: efavirenz, emtricitabine, and tenofovir.

These three drugs are among the preferred first-line recommendations of the HIV treatment guidelines by the U.S. Department of Health and Human Services. Atripla also fits the requirements set out by the International AIDS Society-USA. As a patient, I appreciate the convenience of a three-in-one pill that's taken once a day.

The best medicine always rises to the top. After twenty-five years—rising through the filter of pharmaceutical companies, doctors, treatment experts, and patients—a handful of particular HIV drugs have proved themselves over time. These drugs must be combined in very specific ways.

Tenofovir and emtricitabine are part of the nucleoside class

Technically speaking, nucleosides are actually a class of drugs called *nucleoside reverse transcriptase inhibitors,* sometimes shortened to just *NRTI.* I am going to refer to this class simply as *nukes.* The nukes are the oldest and most-studied class of HIV drugs. The very first HIV drug was called *zidovudine,* or *AZT.*

HIV drugs have improved dramatically since the early days of AZT. Back then, doctors didn't know the best approach was to combine three separate HIV drugs. Instead, they gave higher and higher doses of a single drug, usually AZT. Before the "AIDS cocktail" had been discovered, HIV medicine got a bad reputation because of toxic side effects.

Today, two widely used nukes are called *tenofovir* (which also goes by the brand name Viread) and *emtricitabine* (band name *Emtriva*). Over the years, tenofovir has become preferred over AZT as one ingredient in a first-line combination. Tenofovir is a good drug in terms of effectiveness with few bad side effects. One side effect, however, is that the drug is tough on your kidneys, especially if you if you have a pre-existing kidney condition.

Nukes can be used alone or with other nukes

Generic name	Brand name
abacavir	Ziagen
didanosine	Videx EC
emtricitabine	Emtriva
lamivudine	Epivir
stavudine	Zerit
tenofovir	Viread
zidovudine or AZT	Retrovir

Another member of the nuke family is emtricitabine (pronounced "em-trissit-a-bean"). This drug is basically a chemical clone—also called a "me-too" drug—of another older chemical by name of *lamivudine* (which now goes by its brand name *Epivir*). The advantage of lamivudine and emtricitabine are that they cause other nukes—namely tenofovir and zidovudine—to work even better. But the advantage of emtricitabine over lamivudine is that it has a longer half-life. So if you forget a dose, lamudine is gone faster, while emtricitabine lasts longer in your body.

Three drugs in the nuke class—tenofovir, emtricitabine, and lamivudine—can be used to treat chronic hepatitis B infection. For people with HIV and HBV co-infection, taking these medicines should be carefully considered. Some drugs in the nuke class—namely stavudine (Zerit) and didanosine (Videx EC)—are being used less often because of toxic side effects.

Efavirenz is the most popular non-nucleoside

Of the non-nukes, one is very potent, and another one is safe for pregnant women. The most potent non-nuke is *efavirenz* (pronounced "eff-ah-vir-enz"), which goes by the brand name *Sustiva*. Over the years, efavirenz has performed well, proving to be safe and effective with relatively few major side effects. However, one more-common but less-severe side effect of efavirenz is cloudy thinking or unusual dreams.

"For somebody who already has a sleep disorder or an anxiety problem," says Daniel Berger, M.D., "using Sustiva (efavirenz) wouldn't be the best drug for that individual." For women, it's important to remember that efavirenz may potentially cause genetic defects in unborn children.

I've taken efavirenz for over seven years. I experience the fuzzy-thinking effect. For example, if I take efavirenz in the morning instead of before bed, I can drive and work just fine. But for the first few hours, and for whatever reason, it takes more concentration to make a decision. At its worst, I feel like a character in a Picasso painting.

Non-nukes cannot be used together

Generic name	Brand name
efavirenz	Sustiva
nevirapine	Viramune

Another non-nuke is actually the oldest and it's called *nevirapine*. One brand name in the U.S. is Viramune. Nevirapine didn't perform well in early tests. It wasn't until efavirenz came along that non-nukes enjoyed a boost in popularity. Ultimately, nevirapine was widely studied in developing countries and became useful to prevent transmission of HIV from a pregnant woman to her new child. In the United States, sometimes a short course of nevirapine is used in pregnant women. The most common side effect of nevirapine is a skin rash, which develops in about 25 percent of people taking the drug. On rare occasions, this rash can become much a much worse condition, one that can be fatal.

Ritonavir and atazanavir are key drugs in the protease inhibitor class

In the 1990s, the *protease inhibitor* class of drugs was considered a breakthrough in HIV medicine. The term *AIDS cocktail* was coined by the media to describe combining three drugs from at least two drug classes into one regimen. Protease inhibitors used in combination were what tipped HIV medicine for the better.

Protease inhibitors are potent. They're extremely effective at reducing HIV levels. With time and more usage, problems with protease inhibitors emerged. Some of the problems were pills-per-dose and metabolic abnormalities. In the 1990s, one protease inhibitor required people to take—literally—a dozen pills a day, on top of other HIV drugs. And, although it took years to identify, protease inhibitors often cause high cholesterol, heart problems, and body-shape changes.

Some protease inhibitors are a boost for other drugs

Generic name	Brand name
amprenavir	Agenerase
atazanavir	Reyataz
darunavir	Prezista
fosamprenavir	Lexiva
indinavir	Crixivan
lopinavir + ritonavir	Kaletra
nelfinavir	Viracept
ritonavir	Norvir
saquinavir	Invirase
tipranavir	Aptivus

Ritonavir is an older protease inhibitor, one that by itself, has fallen out of favor. Instead, doctors now use a lower dose to make other protease inhibitors work better. This happens because ritonavir is *hepatically metabolized,* which means that your liver filters your blood. Ritonavir is difficult to filter, so it essentially clogs up in the liver, causing the levels of other drugs in your blood to rise. If you take too many drugs that are hepatically metabolized, your liver can't work fast enough to quickly remove them. Again, this is like the way that algae builds up in a fish tank with a broken filter. Doctors prescribe ritonavir to boost the levels of other drugs. They made this discovery when a patient taking ritonavir accidentally overdosed on the illicit drug ecstasy. These days, ritonavir is mostly used to boost other protease inhibitors only. This is called *ritonavir-boosted* treatment.

There are newer members of the protease inhibitor class. One new protease inhibitor is called atazanavir (brand name Reyataz). The drug is popular because it appears to have less effect on cholesterol and metabolic abnormalities. Doctors often add a low dose of ritonavir to boost the effectiveness of atazanavir. Be aware that protease inhibitors can be hard on your liver, so your doctor should carefully monitor the health of your liver.

First-line HIV medicine means combining three different HIV drugs

According to guidelines by the U.S. Department of Health and Human Services (DHHS) and the International AIDS Society-USA (ISA), a first-line HIV medicine should include "preferred" combinations of drugs. Those preferred drugs can be from any of the three classes, but not all three at any one time. Using just the handful of preferred drugs, there's still a staggering number of potential combinations. Both the DHHS and the ISA guidelines agree that for drug-naïve patients, there are two preferred regimens, one is nuke based, while the other is protease inhibitor based. Here's is a summary:

NON-NUKE-BASED REGIMEN

Two *nukes* plus one *non-nuke*:

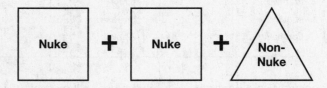

PROTEASE INHIBITOR-BASED REGIMEN

Two *nukes* plus a *boosted protease inhibitor*:

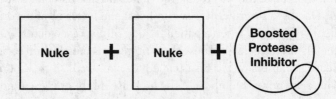

In building a three-drug combination, some combinations and some pairs are preferred over others. Some of those preferred combinations include:

○ tenofovir and emtricitabine (when paired together in one pill, the name is Truvada)
○ tenofovir, emtricitabine, and efavirenz (when all three are combine into one pill, the brand name is Atripla)
○ zidovudine and lamivudine (when paired together in one pill, the name is Combivir)
○ atazanavir and ritonavir (in a boosted regimen)

The future of HIV medicine is bright

Let's be clear: the purpose of taking HIV pills is to save your life. Remember, having a pulse is good. After that, it helps when the medicine is convenient.

Still, HIV medicine improves all the time. "That's the good news and the bad news," says Dr. Fauci. "If you had two million [HIV] copies and 75 [T-cells], I'd grab you by the ears and shake you, 'you really need to be on therapy.' But if you had undetectable virus and 800 [T-cells], I'd say you're absolutely crazy for going on therapy. But, in the same breath, I'd say that you need to follow your [T-cells] and follow your viral load."

Looking down the road of HIV medicine, new drugs within old classes may prove to have fewer side effects. Even entirely new classes of drugs are in development. "More and better" HIV drugs is the direction that HIV medicine is heading, according to Dr. Fauci. "On the horizon are binding, fusion, and entry inhibitors."

Bob Munk, a respected patient expert, concurs that new classes of drugs are on the horizon. However, he hopes the direction of leans toward "more forgiving" drugs. "What are the long-term side effects of these new classes of drugs?" says Munk. "No drug ever looks better than the day it gets approved by the FDA. Great, we've got entry and fusion inhibitors. What does somebody look like after five years on a fusion inhibitor? We won't know until we get there."

IN A SENTENCE:

> *There are several good medicines to construct a safe and effective first-line treatment for HIV.*

living

Managing Coinfection with Hepatitis C and Hepatitis B

WHEN ASKED about managing HIV and viral hepatitis, Anthony Fauci, M.D. advises people to think carefully about secondary diseases. "Have a great familiarity not only with each disease itself, but also with the overlapping and confounding issues of each treatment."

This overlap is seen in a new study that found that the number of deaths due to HCV (in form of death from liver failure or cancer) rose from about 3,700 in the year 1998 and is expected to peak at about 13,000 in the year 2030. In contrast, the same study found that death due to HIV (in the form of immune depletion) was 14,400 in the year 1998 and is expected to dip to 4,200 by the year 2030.

In the U.S., the prevalence of HCV among people with HIV is estimated to be 15 to 30 percent, according to the U.S. Centers of Disease Control and Prevention.

HCV and HIV can influence each other's progression

HCV tends to be more serious in people who have HIV. In some ways, each virus helps the other to survive. For example,

HCV generally damages your liver slowly over time, but it happens more quickly in people with HIV. And with a damaged liver, you can't take HIV medicine.

For people with HCV and HIV, the question becomes: Which virus is the biggest threat to my health? Long-standing HCV disease may lead to development of fibrosis, cirrhosis, liver failure, and liver cancer. One study found that the estimated time from initial HCV infection to cirrhosis in people with HIV was less than the general population. If you grab a hundred HCV-positive people and put them into a room, you find the following averages over time:

- 55–85 of people might develop long-term infection
- 70 people might develop chronic liver disease
- 5–20 people might develop cirrhosis over a period of twenty to thirty years
- 1–5 people might die from the consequences of long term infection, such as liver cancer or cirrhosis
- 10–15 people will spontaneously convert to HCV-negative without treatment at all

At one time, researchers had hoped that HIV treatment *alone* would boost the immune system to eradicate HCV. But it didn't work out that way. In one study, people with both HIV and HCV received HIV medicine for a year. While T-cells and HIV viral load improved with HIV medicine, the levels of HCV were unchanged. The researchers concluded that HIV medicine *by itself* will not lead to better control of HCV replication.

"Treat the HIV first, so you can treat the HCV later," says Cyril Gaultier, M.D. You need to fix the immune system first with HIV medicine in order to get an optimal response from HCV treatment. If your T-cells are high, then you'll have a better chance of success with HCV treatment. "But if your T-cells are below 300 or 400, I would worry about getting the T-cells higher and making the immune system stronger."

Another worry is the bad effects that HIV medicine have on your liver. But Dr. Gaultier notes it really depends on the level of liver damage and the strength of the immune system. "Traditionally we think of lopinavir + ritronavir (Kaletra), efavirenz (Sustiva), and nelfinavir (Viracept) as being safe with HCV."

Three things you can do right now to protect your liver:

1. Stop drinking alcohol

Alcohol (some drugs) are a major assault on your liver. Research on HIV and HCV co-infected people shows these people to be more sensitive to "alcoholic and drug-related" liver disease. Research in HIV and HBV co-infection shows the same.

2. Get a vaccination to prevent hepatitis A

Hepatitis A is a common and easily transmitted virus that attacks the liver. The majority of people recover from this virus. However, if your liver is already burdened by other viruses or HIV medicine, getting hepatitis A is the last thing you need. Have your doctor test your blood to check for immunity against hepatitis A. If you don't have immunity get vaccinated.

3. Check your defenses against hepatitis B

You doctor can test your blood and tell if you have adequate immune defense against HBV. If not, get vaccinated to prevent HBV. The HBV vaccination tends to work best in people with higher T-cell counts. There is a vaccine that protects you against both hepatitis A and B. Although there is no vaccine for HCV, there are ways to avoid catching it

Treatment for HCV is composed of two medicines

Treatment for chronic HCV usually involves two drugs: one is called *alpha interferon* and the other is called *ribavirin*. The interferon part must be injected just below the skin, while the ribavirin part is swallowed as pills: one injection of interferon per week and several pills a day. Side effects are headache, fever, swelling, general pain (and specifically right where you jab the needle). Then there's crankiness and depression, which happens about one quarter of who use interferon. Your doctor should know if the treatment will work within the first twelve weeks.

"I tell people to think about committing a year of their lives to treating HCV—six months if they're lucky to have a nice genotype," says Dr. Gaultier. "And don't underestimate the potential side effects of these drugs." He suggests that people have a good support group. For depression or suicidal thoughts, he offers patients pre-emptive antidepressants. "Wellbutrin works well in those settings. I've found Wellbutrin to be perfect for the interferon blues."

Interferon is a natural protein that your immune system secretes to help fight viruses, bacteria, parasites and cancer cells. In the 1970s, scientists found a way to produce a man-made version of interferon. In the 1980s, researchers tested interferon against HIV. It didn't work well. With further testing, they found that interferon helps boost the immune system. With HIV, there's no immune system to boost, so interferon works best in people with a full immune system. As such, interferon can be helpful in treating other viruses such as HCV, HBV, HPV, and certain forms of cancer. In 2001, the FDA approved a *pegylated interferon* (which means that the interferon is chemically tweaked so it stays in your body longer, requiring only one injection per week).

The story of the drug ribavirin, is one of good and bad marketing. Ribavirin is in the nucleoside class. In the 1970s, it was tested against certain strains of flu with limited success. It wasn't until the late 1990s that doctors found that it boosted the effects of interferon for HCV—just enough to get it approved by the FDA. Since that time, however, the patent ran short and the drug was chemically cloned by different pharmaceutical companies to pair with their own brand of interferon. Whether the pills are called Copegus, Rebetol, Virazole, or RibaSphere, your body only gets ribavirin. Don't forget that sometimes ribavirin interacts with HIV medicine in harmful ways.

CURRENTLY, TREATMENT with pegylated interferon plus ribavirin is the standard treatment of HCV in HIV-positive people and the only FDA-approved treatment for co-infection.

HCV treatment has two parts: interferon and ribavirin

Generic name	Brand name
peginterferon alfa-2a + ribavirin	Pegasys + Copegus
pegylated interferon alfa-2b + ribavirin	PEG-Intron + Rebetol

The National Institutes of Health issued a consensus statement on managing HCV. The following recommendations were made for when and how to treat HCV among the general population:

Medicine to treat HCV

For Genotype 1:
Treat with pegylated interferon + ribavirin for forty-eight weeks

For Genotype 2 or 3:

Treat with pegylated interferon + ribavirin

or

Standard interferon + ribavirin for twenty-four weeks

When to treat HCV

The time to treat is when HCV viral load exceeds 50 IU/mL

plus

Liver biopsy shows portal or bridging fibrosis and at least moderate inflammation

plus

No active injection drug use, alcoholism, neuropsychiatric disorder, or decompensated liver disease. (Anxiety and depression are examples of neuropsychiatric disorders while cirrhosis—or scar tissue—is an example of decompensated liver disease).

In people with HIV and HCV co-infection, the duration of HCV treatment is usually forty-eight weeks, regardless of HCV genotype. However, some doctors are considering eighteen months of treatment for co–infected people who have HCV genotype 1. The primary goal of HCV treatment is sustained virological response (SVR) which is no detectable HCV in the blood in the six months after end of therapy. Sustained virological response is an indication of long-term remission of HCV, but some experts consider it a cure.

In each case, treatment may be discontinued at 12 weeks if there's not a dramatic decrease in HCV levels. While these guidelines are aimed at the general population, new research has shown that this 12-week decision is valid for HIV-positive people. Research with pegylated interferon plus ribavirin suggest this treatment may have a promising, if limited role, in "clearing" HCV among HIV-HCV co-infected people. They cautioned, however, that side effects and adherence should be closely monitored.

In HCV among the general population, more than 85 percent maintain undetectable HCV levels for up to ten years after completion of HCV treatment. For people with HIV, HCV treatment may help improve the condition of the liver, so it can process HIV medicine.

Managing hepatitis B and HIV has gotten easier

"There are many patients who cannot think about HIV without think-ing about the hepatitis [effects] as well," says Anthony Fauci, M.D. "For HBV, the decision to treat is more complicated because some of the drugs used for fighting HBV are the very same drugs used for fighting HIV."

One class of drugs used for both HIV and HBV are the nukes (nucleo-side reverse transcriptase inhibitors). Years ago, doctors discovered that one nuke, lamivudine, helped fight not only HIV but also HBV. The problem with lamivudine for HBV is that it doesn't work for long. When lamivudine is used for HBV in people co-infected with both viruses, the drug stops working for HBV very quickly.

If you have HIV or HBV, you can still get HCV

JUST BECAUSE you have HIV or HBV, doesn't mean you still can't get hep-atitis C. For years, doctors thought that getting HCV through sexual contact was possible, but unlikely. Now, they are changing their tune. A widely publicized out-break of HCV was discovered among a group of HIV-positive men who often had group sex together. One of them got HCV and they all got HCV. Dr. Gaultier points out that the cause of HCV transmission is really due to rough anal sex without a condom and microscopic blood and abrasions. If you're HIV-positive, there are things you can do to protect yourself:

- ◯ Avoid unprotected anal intercourse without a condom. This applies to women having anal sex with a male partner.
- ◯ Avoid rough-sex practices such as fisting.
- ◯ Don't share sex toys.
- ◯ Avoid sexual activity under the influence of illicit drugs, especially crystal meth.
- ◯ Avoid sharing a straw or rolled-up dollar bill if snorting cocaine.
- ◯ Stop injecting drugs or never start. If you continue to inject drugs, always use clean needles. Don't reuse or share water or drug preparation equipment.
- ◯ Don't share toothbrushes, floss, or razors that might be contaminated with blood.

Adefovir is a nuke that began its career as an HIV drug but found a bet-ter role in treating HBV. For the higher doses needed to fight HIV, the drug caused unacceptable kidney damage and was abandoned for HIV. Instead, its manufacturer sought and received FDA approval to sell adefovir—at much lower doses—to treat HBV.

Tenofovir is another HIV drug with substantial activity against HBV. This is not surprising because tenofovir is chemically similar to adefovir. Today, tenofovir is approved by the FDA to treat HIV only. The research, however, shows that tenofovir is equally if not more effective than adefovir for treating HBV.

The drug emtricitabine (band name Emtriva) is basically a clone of lamivudine. As such, both drugs are about equally effective at treating HBV, which is say that, *by themselves*, both lamivudine and emtricitabine don't work well over the long run for HBV.

Fauci offered a word of caution. The damage that HBV causes to the liver comes mostly from the immune system. With untreated HIV, the immune system is suppressed—so there's less damage being done to the liver. However, if the immune system regains strength with HIV medicine, there's the possibility of a "secondary immune reactivation" also called a "flare" from smoldering HBV infection. This flare can cause some liver damage.

Nukes can be used alone or with other nukes to treat HBV

Generic name	Brand name when used for HIV	Brand name when used for HBV
adefovir	Not used to treat HIV	Hepsera
entecavir	Not used to treat HIV	Baraclude
emtricitabine	Emtriva	About as active against HBV as lamivudine, but not approved by the FDA for HBV
lamivudine	Epivir	Epivir-HBV
telbivudine	Not used to treat HIV	Tyzeka
tenofovir	Viread	Highly active against HBV, but not approved by the FDA for HBV

Still, the future of HIV and HBV co-infection is being worked out very well, according to Dr. Fauci. "In the era of [HIV medicine], the long-range prognosis for people with HIV, in regard to their HIV, has changed so dramatically that it's essential to pay as much attention to other issues that were always far secondary—among those hepatitis is one of the most important."

Liver biopsy is the gold standard for assessing liver damage

Liver biopsies really aren't so scary. Sure, people cringe when I admit to having two liver biopsies—a diagnostic procedure that retrieves a snippet of liver tissue for examination under a microscope. At first, the procedure sounds reasonable, as the results can give you the bottom line on the health of your liver.

What gives people the heebie-jeebies is how doctors actually get the sample. A specialist sticks a long needle between your ribs, piercing your liver. The needle is hollow, so it draws back a thin, long slice of your liver. The needle jab takes only seconds. I didn't feel a thing either time.

In general, liver biopsies are used to check if your liver is scarred (scar tissue is beginning to replace functioning liver cells), if inflammation (cellular infiltration and swelling) is present, or if necrosis (dead liver cells) is present. When the liver becomes permanently injured, it's called *cirrhosis*.

It's possible to get a liver transplant—even if you have HIV

AIDS activist, founder of ACT-UP, and acclaimed writer Larry Kramer got a new liver in 2001. At 66 years of age, and after a widely publicized plea for a liver transplant, Kramer got his wish. These days, he's also got a new soapbox: Cutting the red tape that's involved with organ transplant policy in the United States, most notably for people with HIV. Traditionally, people with HIV are excluded from receiving organ transplants.

"In Kramer's case, his HIV has been relatively well controlled. However, like many HIV patients with viral hepatitis, his liver disease continued to progress in spite of anti-hepatitis medications," says John Fung, M.D., chief of the division of transplant surgery at the University of Pittsburgh School of Medicine (UPMC). "For the most part, results have been good and most of our patients can expect to do well after transplantation."

UPMC is one of ten centers participating in a National Institutes of Health–funded study to determine the safety and effectiveness of liver and kidney transplantation in patients with HIV. The results of this study may be useful to the entire transplant and infectious-disease community as physicians and surgeons attempt to define the best care for people who are co-infected with HIV and viral hepatitis.

IN A SENTENCE:

> *If you have HIV and are co-infected with HCV or HBV, your treatment strategy should consider both infections and the health of your liver, which can be assessed by blood tests or a liver biopsy.*

learning

Metabolic Syndromes and Body-Shape Changes

EARLIER CHAPTERS discussed the benefits of HIV medicine. You should also know about some of the most-common and most-severe side effects. In later chapters, I'll discuss immediate side effects (including nausea when you first begin medicine). This chapter concerns long-term consequences that may take years to notice. These side effects include metabolic syndromes and body-shape changes.

In the past, side effects became so troubling, some people deliberately stopped taking the medicine. For other people, fear of these side effects prevents them from taking the medicine in the first place. "It was one of my first big fears," say Paul T., who tested positive four months ago. "Sunken cheeks are the worst aspect of being 'HIV'. It gives away your HIV status to people. I'm probably more aware of the changes than the average person. Still, in some communities, everybody knows what sunken cheeks mean."

Research suggests that body-fat abnormalities occur in almost half of people taking HIV medicine. Doctors are beginning to find the root cause as *mitochondrial toxicity*, which has been implicated in fat loss from some parts of the body, tumor-like fat accumulation in other parts, abnormally high cholesterol and triglycerides, and diabetes-like problems with blood sugar.

Some nucleosides may kill brown fat

If you've ever taken a biology class, you'd know *mitochondria*. Mitochondria are tiny "organs" that live inside of a larger cell, especially in animal and human cells. Mitochondria are sometimes described as "cellular power plants" because they convert food into energy, and then the energy takes the form of movement or heat.

So it makes sense that higher-than-normal numbers of mitochondria live inside of a typical human fat cell. When you run a mile and you get warm, it's the mitochondria in your cells that are responsible. All human fat cells come two colors: brown and white. Brown fat generates heat in response to cold temperatures or excess caloric intake. Brown fat is plentiful in babies to guard against the cold.

As humans age, most of the mitochondria (which are responsible for the brown color) in brown fat disappear. This is one reason why we lose baby fat as we age. The remaining tissue becomes similar to white fat, what we all know as a belly fat. In humans, white fat composes as much as 20 percent of the body weight in men and 25 percent of the body weight in women. Some adults, however, do retain some brown fat.

Fat loss can happen in different places of the body

In the face—fat loss in the face can occur in the cheeks, temples, and forehead. Facial fat loss is what many call "sunken cheeks."

In the legs, arms, and buttocks—fat loss can occur in the arms and legs. Sometimes this gives people "skinny legs." Other people like the fat loss in the arms because muscles and veins are more noticeable. But fat loss in the buttocks, making a flat butt, distresses some people.

In the HIV community, the term *lipodystrophy* is often used to describe a number of different conditions. The word *lipid* means fat. The word *dystrophy* means shrinking. So the term *lipodystrophy* is accurate for describing the shrinkage of fat in certain areas of you body, but it's technically inaccurate when used to describe the accumulation of fat in other areas. Terms that are more accurate are *lipid abnormalities* or *body-shape changes*.

New research suggests that HIV medicines disrupt, if not permanently kill, the mitochondria inside of brown fat (also called *adipocytes*). "Brown adipocytes could be preferential targets of [HIV-medicine]-induced mito-chondrial toxicity as these cells have a high mitochondrial content, in con-trast with white adipocytes." Research is being conducted on the mitochondria and fat cells, but specifics are not yet known.

However, it is clear that some HIV medicines can be linked to certain types of fat loss. According to Cyril Gaultier, M.D., an infectious disease and HIV specialist in Palm Springs, California, stavudine (Zerit) and didanosine (Videx EC) seem to be the worst in terms of loss of fat in the face, arms, and legs. To a lesser extent long-term use of zidovudine (Retro-vir, AZT) leads to fat loss in the same areas of the body, but it also tends to cause more fat loss in the buttocks.

Daniel Berger, M.D., an HIV specialist in Chicago, notes that there's a pecking order for HIV medicines and their toxicities on mitochondria. "Of the nukes that we use, we know some are not so good and some are better."

Not-so-good nukes

Generic name	Brand name
didanosine	Videx EC
stavudine	Zerit
zidovudine or AZT	Retrovir

Better nukes

Generic name	Brand name
abacavir	Ziagen
emtricitabine	Emtriva
lamivudine	Epivir
tenofovir	Viread

HIV medicines may disrupt various other fat cells

Fat accumulation is called *lipohypertrophy*. Fat accumulation among peo-ple taking HIV medicine can be divided into two categories: tumor-like fatty lumps and belly fat. The tumor-like fat can be lumpy or fatty tissue that often grows below the skin and behind the neck. This is sometimes called *dorsocervical fat pads* or "buffalo hump." A recent study estimated that buf-falo hump happens in around 6 percent of people taking HIV medicine. Researchers speculate that the unusual syndrome has something to do with mitochondria. Instead of killing the fat cells, it causes them to grow out of control and to look more like brown fat cells instead of the white ones.

"There's a lipodystrophy study where people had developed buffalo humps on [the drug] Kaletra and they also had high cholesterol," says Dr. Gaultier. "They were switched to Reyataz and the cholesterol got much lower. And after one year, a lot of the patients actually had a decline in their buffalo hump, suggesting that Reyataz, at least, doesn't fuel buffalo hump. Since we stopped using drugs like Zerit and Videx, the percentage of people who show up with buffalo humps is almost gone."

As for belly fat, also called *abdominal fat* or *abdominal adiposity*, it's quite a different story. Belly fat is your standard-issue fat and it's usually associated with eating too much and not exercising enough. New research suggests that in HIV-positive people, metabolic syndrome rates—including increased belly fat—are equal to the general population, which is about one in four people.

One recent study suggested that prevalence of metabolic syndrome in HIV-positive people may reflect the growing epidemic of obesity, more than the adverse effects of HIV medicine. The risk of "metabolic syndrome in HIV-infected persons is not significantly greater than the risk in HIV-uninfected persons of the same age, race, sex, and smoking status," the researchers noted.

Even so, the researchers still found that specific medications—lopinavir + ritonavir (Kaletra) and didanosine (Videx)—were associated with an increased risk of metabolic syndrome. They cautioned, however, that it's still important to address precursors of heart disease and diabetes.

Fat accumulation can happen in different parts of the body

Deep within the belly—fat growth below the stomach muscles makes the belly protrude but feel hard, not soft and squeezable like normal belly fat.

In the breasts—fat growth in the chest area and enlarged breasts can occur in both men and women (but it's more common in women).

High cholesterol and triglycerides can lead to heart disease

There are different types of fat (also called lipids) that float around in your blood—cholesterol and triglycerides. Of the cholesterol type, there's good and bad cholesterol also called *high-density lipoprotein (HDL)* and *low-density lipoprotein (LDL)*. Triglycerides are a third type of fat known as *fatty acids*. If you have high levels of HDL, that's a good thing. But if you have high levels of LDL or triglycerides, that's bad.

High levels of HDL–good

High levels of LDL–bad

High levels of Triglycerides–bad

Protease inhibitors can cause significant increases in LDL and triglycerides. One protease inhibitor in particular, ritonivir (Norvir), seems to be the worst in terms of elevating LDL and triglycerides. Dr. Gaultier points to the protease inhibitors, lopinavir + ritronavir (Kaletra) and ritonavir-boosted saquinavir (Invirase) as the worst offenders.

Doctors suspect that mitochondria toxicity plays a role in increasing LDL and triglycerides as well. Whatever the cause, the abnormalities do contribute to risk for heart disease and stroke. If you already have higher than normal LDL or triglyceride levels, or if you have pre-existing heart conditions, if someone in your family has heart conditions—an HIV regimen containing a protease inhibitor might not be best for you.

Not-so-good protease inhibitors

Generic name	Brand name
indinavir	Crixivan
lopinavir + ritronavir	Kaletra
ritonavir	Norvir
saquinavir	Invirase

Better protease inhibitors

Generic name	Brand name
atazanavir	Reyataz
darunavir	Prezista

Some HIV medicines cause blood sugar problems and diabetes

Insulin is a hormone made by the pancreas to help the cells in your body absorb a sugar called *glucose*. *Insulin resistance* is when the cells your body refuse to accept insulin. When this happens, the levels of insulin in the blood become dangerously high, eventually leading to *Type 2 diabetes*. In general, insulin resistance is involved with heart disease, blood abnormalities, fat metabolism, and blood pressure.

About 40 percent of people who take a protease inhibitor will have abnormal glucose levels due to insulin resistance. Doctors know that protease inhibitors play a key role, but exactly how is still not clear. One specific protease inhibitor called indinavir (Crixivan) is strongly linked to the condition.

Do protease inhibitors cause glucose metabolism problems? "Yes, in some patients, but not in everyone,"says Dr. Berger. "Most protease inhibitors cause some types of problems or insulin resistance or diabetes-like problems. When you stop the protease inhibitors, often those symptoms improve. This is proof that, in some individuals, protease inhibitors are the culprit."

Berger offers the following tips if you are considering a protease inhibitor:

○ Be sure your physician is aware of potential side effects, including diabetes or insulin resistance. You might be surprised to learn than some doctors may not be aware of these side effects.

○ Have what's called a *glucose tolerance test*. You arrive at your doctor's office having not eaten. You'll get a blood test before you drink a liquid with glucose in it. Two hours later, you'll get another blood test. The results help you and your doctor decide if insulin resistance is a problem.

○ Consider your family history of diabetes.

○ Take into account your body-fat composition. If you're very overweight, you're at a much higher risk for diabetes.

○ Exercise and good dietary judgment can change the course of diabetes and insulin resistance.

○ Be vigilant about monitoring.

Diet and exercise can improve or prevent body shape changes

If you start HIV medicine and encounter elevations in LDL or triglycerides, you have options. First is changing your diet. Eat less, eat better, and reduce alcohol consumption, all of which lead to weight loss. Although the International AIDS Society suggests that the Mediterranean diet improves heart health, there is no consensus about the role of a specialized diet for people with body shape changes—unless other metabolic abnormalities or weight loss is also a consideration. Still, the organization points out that it's prudent to reduce intake of saturated fat, simple carbohydrates, and alcohol.

Another option is aerobic and resistance exercise. The approach has been shown effective as a non-chemical intervention for abdominal fat buildup. Moderate exercise is well tolerated in people with HIV and does not increase viral load.

You can avert many problems being active, exercising, and making good dietary habits, says Berger. "Athletes are less likely to have the body-shape problems. I have patients who are professional athletes and dancers, and I can't think of one instance of body-shape problems with them, regardless of what protease inhibitor they're taking."

We know from research that exercise and diet plays a role in diabetes treatment and prevention. We know that exercise by itself can reduce fat accumulation in people with HIV. Being overweight is bad for your health in general. Fat accumulation can cause glucose and heart problems. Exercise reduces glucose problems. It's just common sense that people considering HIV medicine should also consider improving diet and exercise habits.

Hormones, steroids, or testosterone are ways to combat body shape changes

Over the years, I've seen a lot of people use a lot of things to gain muscle and lose fat. Years ago, *AIDS wasting* was the big problem among the HIV community. *Wasting* is significant loss of lean body mass due to major illness. Back then, pharmaceutical companies hyped testosterone, anabolic steroids, and human growth hormone to improve lean body mass. After all, studies do show testosterone, anabolic steroids, and human growth hormone are helpful for wasting.

One brand of human growth hormone called *Serostim* is approved by the FDA as a treatment for AIDS wasting. Serostim will likely get FDA approval for "lipo-accumulation" caused by HIV medicine. Besides being expensive as a drug, it has serious side effects, including causing diabetes, fluid retention, joint aches, and carpal tunnel syndrome.

Another approach to growth hormone is called *human growth hormone releasing factor,* which is a hormone produced by a gland in the brain. What sets it apart from regular growth hormone is that the body's system of regulating levels of the hormone are still in-tact with the releasing factor. This may be a way to avoid the toxicity normally associated with standard growth hormone treatment.

Testosterone is a weapon against wasting and helps improve lean body mass. Testosterone is important for bone mineralization, cognitive functioning, and averting depression. For men with low testosterone, replacement of testosterone might be considered. Some people with HIV also use anabolic steroids to help combat body-shape changes. Whether or not your doctor prescribes anabolic steroids, it's important to at least inform your doctor that you are using steroids.

According to Dr. Gaultier, it's important to know the *whole* story when it comes to anabolic steroids. He offers a few considerations about using steroids:

ANABOLIC STEROIDS ARE TOUGH ON YOUR LIVER

Anabolic steroids should be prescribed with great caution in people with HIV and hepatitis co-infection. These drugs can cause problems with your liver's ability to process drugs. They can also cause liver damage, which might require an interruption of the HIV medicine. Oral anabolic steroids are more likely to affect the liver than injectable formulations, such as *decadurabulin.*

LONG-TERM USE OF ANABOLIC STEROIDS CAN LEAD TO HEART ATTACKS

Long-term use leads to lower levels of good cholesterol (also called HDL) and higher levels of bad cholesterol (also called LDL). Normal HDL should be over 45 and with anabolic use, HDL commonly drops to with the 10-to-20 range. This leads to increased risk of *cholesterol plaques* in the heart, which can then lead to heart attacks.

LONG-TERM USE OF ANABOLIC STEROIDS ALSO DEFORMS THE HEART

Anabolic steroids do make your biceps bigger, but they also make your heart muscles grow as well. This can cause your heart to become too muscular and too big, which ultimately weakens your heart. This happens because the bigger heart has less room for the inner chambers needed to pump blood. There's no room inside of your heart for blood to be pumped out. This can lead to heart failure.

USE ANABOLIC STEROIDS ONLY WITH MEDICAL SUPERVISION

As a whole, anabolic steroids should be used under close medical supervision with attention to the liver, cholesterol levels, and the heart. For HIV and AIDS, anabolics can be used for AIDS wasting, which is defined as a 10 percent loss of body weight (but primarily muscle mass). Special caution to those who discontinue anabolic steroids after many years of use. These people should taper the doses over time to avoid withdrawal syndromes.

IN A SENTENCE:

> *HIV medicine can cause problems with fat cells in your body, but there are ways to reduce or avoid the problems.*

MONTH **10**

Taking HIV Medicine Every Day: An Action Plan

RESEARCH ON human behavior shows that radical behavior changes are rarely sustained over time. Of course, you *can* change your behavior for a while, but it's hard to stick with it over time. Therefore, some people "slip" or "cheat" and then feel guilty, which usually leads to even more problematic behaviors.

We are human beings, not machines. We're imperfect, emotional, and generally prefer pleasure to pain. Sticking to HIV medicine—as prescribed—is not that different from sticking to a diet or an exercise plan. You may know *what* to do, *why* it's important, and *how* to do it, but actually *doing it* over the long term doesn't always pan out.

The motivation to take your HIV medicine every day in the right way *must* come from within you. You are the master of your health. You have a choice: Either take the pills or don't. But remember, every choice you make has consequences for you and for others. Here are a few considerations should you choose to begin HIV medicine.

What it means to be adherent

Doctors define *adherence* as the "extent to which a patient's behavior corresponds with medical advice." This can include whether you keep your appointments, following up if the doctor refers you to another doctor or specialist, following your doctor's advice about health-related suggestions, and taking medicine according to the prescribed dosage, frequency, timing, and food requirements. The term *non-adherence* means "not" doing these things. From here on, let's just focus on adherence to HIV medicine.

Better adherence means better response to HIV medicine. However, let's take a closer look at what this means in real life. First you need to understand what *resistant virus* means. HIV becomes *resistant* when it learns how to *resist* one more HIV drugs. When this happens, the virus no longer responds to any medicine—and that's bad.

Research shows that taking your meds less than 50 percent of the time does not lead to resistant virus. That's because the levels of the drug are so low, there's very little pressure on the virus to change. So what happens is the virus continues to multiply and gobble up your T-cells, unfazed by this half-hearted effort to stop it.

On the other hand, if you take your HIV medicine more than 95 percent of the time, resistant virus also does not develop. The reason for this is because the virus is basically snuffed out so completely that it can't develop resistance. There's essentially no virus around to become resistant. No virus, no resistance.

The big problem comes into play when people are between 70 and 95 percent adherent to medicine. In this range, enough of the drugs are in your body to put pressure on the virus. If there's not enough pressure to snuff out the virus entirely, some of it will survive. The virus that survives is resistant and it's especially nasty because it will forever know how to get around any HIV medicine. Eventually, this resistant HIV will grow and replace the original virus (called "wild type virus").

The lesson: you need to be more than 95 percent adherent to keep the virus at bay for the long run. But what does this mean in your everyday life? Let's look at the actual numbers:

ONCE-A-DAY REGIMEN
Goal: 95 percent adherence
This means you could miss 1.5 doses a month (30 days) and still be okay. Since you have to do better than 95 percent, round it up and say you could miss one dose. This means you could miss a dose once a month and not

develop resistance. If you were to miss two doses per month, you'd be at around 93 percent adherent—not good enough. Missing three doses a month, you would be about 90 percent adherent. Remember, anything less than 95 percent puts you at high risk for developing resistant HIV.

TWICE-A-DAY REGIMEN
Goal: 95 percent adherence

A twice a day regimen is a little more forgiving because you could miss three doses a month and probably be okay. But remember, that's three *doses* not three *days*. If you think in terms of days, you could miss one and a half days and still be okay. But don't fool yourself, missing three doses in a row is worse than missing one dose a day over the span of weeks. It doesn't mean you can take a weekend off from you meds.

Get to know yourself before you begin medicine

You're probably thinking: "No problem, I could easily take my medicine every day," with the caveat that you have a "spare day" in case you forget. Well, let's put your thoughts into action. Here's a simple at-home test to assess your own level of adherence:

1. Purchase a thirty-day supply of once-a-day vitamins. It doesn't matter what kind of vitamins, anything that fits your budget or preference. However, it's important that there be exactly 30 pills.
2. Get a calendar and count out exactly 30 days. Take note of your beginning date and your end date.
3. Write your "beginning date" and your "end date" directly on the bottle of vitamins. Now begin taking one vitamin once a day.
4. In one month from now, when you reach the "end day," check the bottle to see how many vitamins are left over.
5. Now, score yourself against the number of pills that remain in the bottle:

   ○ **one pill**: Congratulations, you're doing better than 95 percent.
   ○ **two pills**: This means you're scoring at about 93 percent, which is pretty good.
   ○ **three pills**: Here you're right at 90 percent adherent. You're on the right track. Think about why you missed those three doses and consider how you can do better.

O   **more than three pills**: Anything more than three pills leftover
means you're scoring at less than 90 percent. Unfortunately, with
HIV medicine you'll either need to achieve 95 percent adherence
or not take the medicine at all.

Obviously, the results of this simple test should not make or break your
decision to begin HIV medicine. But it will help you get a sense of what it
takes to be better than 95 percent adherent in the real world. If you're scoring at less than 90 percent, think seriously about what's going on in your
life that's preventing you from taking the pills. If you managed to get
through the month and missed one dose or less, adherence is unlikely to
be a problem for you.

IN A SENTENCE:

> *A simple test will help you understand what it means to be better
> than 95 percent adherent to your HIV medicine.*

learning

Your First HIV Pill: Short-Term Side Effects

I CLEARLY recall swallowing the first pills of my three-drug combination. I remember thinking they seemed like an awful lot of pills to take at one time.

With a glass of water, they went down easily enough. An hour went by and I felt nothing. A few more hours went by and still, I didn't feel a thing. Then came time for my second dose, and again, no problems. Nothing at all. I thought, this is going to be a breeze—for about one week. Then it hit me: a wave of nausea washed over me while on the bus headed to work. The nausea persisted. I remember walking past a Starbucks and the smell gave me the dry heaves.

For about two more weeks, my mouth tasted like I was sucking on a dirty penny. The whites of my eyes didn't quite seem white. I felt toxic. I dreaded "pill time" because I knew it translated to several hours of queasiness, hardly a motivator for me.

Finally, I couldn't take it any longer. I called my doctor and said "uncle." I give up. I couldn't imagine feeling like this forever. His response? "Well, your T-cells doubled and your viral load is undetectable." With that, everything changed.

With time, the side effects subsided almost completely. With more time, my T-cells tripled and quadrupled. And I haven't seen a viral load above 40 copies since 1996.

Expect some degree of short-term side effects when you first start HIV treatment. Sure, you may be lucky and sneak by without any side effects at all. On the other hand, you may be that one-in-one-hundred person that winds up with a medical rarity. The key is knowing what's normal and what's not. Nausea and diarrhea are common events and will go away with time. Rash and fever, however, can be red flags for more serious situations. It's a good idea to write down any symptoms in a health journal so you can describe them in detail to your doctor and remember what drugs may be causing side effects.

If you begin to experience intolerable side effects, be aggressive with your doctor about communicating your symptoms. Remember, only in rare cases are side effects serious enough to require medical attention. Above all, don't just *not* take your medicine because you're going to a party later or because you just don't feel like it. Know that your side effects will subside with time. Down the road, you will get the rewards of better health and a longer life.

Side effects vary greatly from person to person

"Side effects? Nope, I didn't have any, thank God," says Precious J., a treatment advocate for Women Alive, an AIDS service organization in Los Angeles, California. For Tim L., the story couldn't be any more different. "As the new meds came out, I tried each one of them because I had so many side effects. I didn't last more than twenty days on any of them," says Tim L.

"I finally tried Viracept with other meds," says Tim L. "That combination seemed to work. The only side effect at first was diarrhea, but I got that under control with [an anti-diarrhea drug called Lomotil]. Once I adjusted to it, I could maintain things without too many problems. Ninety percent of the time, the diarrhea is under control. Once in awhile I'll get diarrhea, so I'll take more Lomotil. I had some nausea at first. I still have gas, but it's one of those things you learn to live with."

Don't worry about all the side effects—just the most common and most severe

First thing, before you take your meds, ask your doctor:

○ What are the *most common* side effects of *all* your meds?
○ What are the *most severe* side effects for *all* your meds?

Remember, you'll be taking at least three different drugs and each one has potentially dozens of side effects. It's probably a waste of time to learn about every side effect for every drug. Instead, focus on the *most common* and the *most severe* ones.

Remember, what's true for the majority may not be true for the individual. Your genetics, your gender, your diet, your lifestyle, co-infections, and just plain luck make you different from the next person. The way your body metabolizes HIV medicine may be different from how somebody else's body might react.

Studies show that women sometimes experience different, more frequent, and more severe side effects than men. This may be due to the fact that women generally weigh less than men do, but they're usually required to take the same amount of drug. Another possible reason might be hormonal differences between genders.

Many people have an adjustment period when starting HIV medicine. This lasts about four to six weeks while your body adapts to the new drug. During this time, you may have headaches, nausea, muscle pain, or occasional dizziness. These kinds of side effects usually lessen or disappear with time. Don't forget that some side effects may actually be due to anxiety, depression, or stress. Keep your emotions and thoughts in check during the adjustment period.

Consider making the adjustment period easier by taking some time off work or lightening your schedule. See if someone can help around the house or help with children.

Here are some common side effects you'll likely experience and a few ways to manage them:

HEADACHE

Headache is a very common side effect of HIV medicine. Expect headaches during the adjustment period. Most times, headaches can be eased by over-the-counter medications like aspirin, acetaminophen, ibuprofen, or naproxen sodium. But check with your doctor beforehand to make sure there are no interactions between these drugs and your HIV medicine.

For instant relief from a throbbing head, try resting in a quiet, dark room with your eyes closed. Place a cold washcloth over your eyes. Massage the base of your skull with your thumbs and massage both temples gently, or try a hot bath.

Anticipate when the pain will strike. Avoid or limit foods known to trigger headaches, especially caffeine (from coffee, tea, soft drinks, or some medications), chocolate, food additives (like monosodium glutamate, or MSG), nuts, onions, hard cheese, and vinegar.

NAUSEA AND VOMITING

Nausea and the urge to vomit are absolutely awful feelings. Understand that this side effect is common and will eventually subside. Persistent vomiting, however, can lead to serious medical problems, such as dehydration, chemical imbalances, or damage to your throat. Call your doctor if you vomit repeatedly throughout the day or if vomiting persists or interferes with your ability to keep down your meds.

The BRAT diet—**B**ananas, **R**ice, **A**pplesauce, and **T**oast—can help with nausea and diarrhea. Try some peppermint, chamomile, or ginger tea—they can calm the stomach.

Sip cold carbonated drinks like ginger ale or 7-Up. Avoid hot, spicy, strong-smelling, and greasy foods. If vomiting occurs, replenish fluids with broth, apple juice, Jell-O, popsicles, or Gatorade.

If nausea or vomiting still persists, don't hesitate to ask your doctor for anti-nausea medications such as compazine or Marinol—they can help immensely.

DIARRHEA

Diarrhea is extremely annoying, extremely common, but also very manageable. If you experience persistent diarrhea, first replenish lost liquids by drinking plenty of fluids, like Gatorade, ginger ale, chicken or beef broth, herb tea, or just plain water. The BRAT diet can help somewhat with this side effect.

Try anti-diarrhea medications like Lomotil, Kaopectate, Immodium, or Pepto-Bismol. Take as prescribed on the package. Eat foods high in soluble fiber, which slows diarrhea by absorbing liquid. In addition to the BRAT diet, these foods include oatmeal, cream of wheat, grits, and soft bread (not whole grain).

• • •

Avoid foods high in insoluble fiber, like the skins of vegetables and fruits. These foods can make diarrhea worse. Avoid milk products and greasy, high-fiber, or very sweet foods. They tend to aggravate diarrhea.

Fatigue

Fatigue is a little more than garden-variety tiredness. Fatigue is a more profound tiredness that keeps you from doing the normal things in life and it's common during the adjustment period. You may feel weary or exhausted in a physical, emotional, or mental way. Your body, especially your arms and legs, may feel heavy. You may find it hard to concentrate or think clearly.

Rest and sleep are important, but don't sleep too much, this can decrease your energy level. In other words, the more you rest, the more tired you will feel. If you have trouble sleeping, talk to your doctor or nurse. Consider taking a "power nap" during the day for one hour or less.

Stay as active as you can. Try light exercise such as walking. You may find that you're most able to exercise early in the day. Try spreading your activities throughout the day. Let others help you with meals, housework, or errands.

If fatigue persists longer than four to six weeks, ask your doctor about anemia. Anemia means the blood has a low red blood cell count, and red blood cells are the vehicles that deliver oxygen to different parts of your body. When your body is short on oxygen, you feel fatigued. The HIV drug zidovudine or AZT (Retrovir) is notorious for causing anemia, especially in women.

Doctors are usually quick to dismiss fatigue as "something in your head," stress, or depression. If it persists, you'll need to become more assertive with your health-care provider. If you are writing down symptoms in your health journal, you will be better able to describe in detail how fatigue is interfering with normal activities and ask specifically about your red blood cell count. There are treatments for both fatigue and anemia.

Allergic drug reactions

Abacavir (Ziagen)

About 3 to 5 percent of people who take the drug abacavir (Ziagen) have a potentially serious allergic reaction to it. This usually develops within two weeks of starting the drug. However, it can appear up to six weeks or more after starting. Signs of this reaction include fever, rash, cough, shortness of breath, or sore throat. If you develop any of these symptoms while taking abacavir, call your doctor immediately.

If you have an allergic reaction to abacavir, do not ever start taking it again. A few allergic patients who re-started abacavir had life-threatening reactions. If you ever stopped abacavir for any reason (for example, because you ran out), talk to your doctor before you start again. In rare cases, people who thought they weren't allergic had serious reactions when re-starting abacavir.

NEVIRAPINE (VIRAMUNE)

The most common side effect with nevirapine is skin rash, which occurs among 17 percent of patients who take the drug. The majority of severe rashes occurred within the first month of taking nevirapine. Most rashes are mild-to-moderate, but can be severe or life-threatening. If you develop any rash-like symptoms while taking nevirapine, contact your physician immediately, or go to an emergency room.

Every so often, side effects can become serious enough—or annoying enough—to require a switch one or more of the drugs in your combination. Switching a drug solely because of side effects may also save that drug as an option future. In fact, side effects from a drug at one time may not occur again if you take the drug later.

Believe me. I know how miserable it is when you're on the edge of vomiting all day long. It's not fun and it changes your entire outlook on life. Some days, it can feel as if life isn't worth living. But it is worth living and you'll put yourself in a really bad spot down the road by simply stopping one drug in your combination, or reducing the dose without talking first with your doctor and pharmacist.

On the bright side, there's good news: The preferred HIV medicines are greatly improved over older ones. The preferred HIV drugs—these drugs—have very little immediate side effects.

IN A SENTENCE:

> *You should expect some side effects from HIV treatment, but they'll likely subside with time.*

living

How to Know if HIV Medicine Is Failing

A RISING viral load while on HIV treatment usually means one of three things: (1) your drug combination isn't working anymore, (2) you're not adhering to the drug combination, or (3) you're experiencing a "viral blip," a transient and temporary rise of viral load that's common and doesn't mean anything. The problem is that all three scenarios start off in the same fashion—your viral load begins to rise despite HIV medicine.

First off, don't panic. If you're on HIV medicine and you get *one* viral load test that's higher than expected, it may not mean a whole lot. However, if you get two or three viral load results that consistently show an increase, that's a different story.

It's true that sometime during your treatment lifetime you may fail HIV medicine—or—the HIV medicine will fail you. It happens both ways. Either way, there are still other options. You may need to switch some drugs around. You may need to adhere to your meds with more vigilance. You don't want to let the situation spiral out of control, which ultimately leads to more loss of immune function.

You'll have more options and more peace of mind by knowing your treatment options down the road. Imagine driving on an unfamiliar highway with only a half tank of gas. One option is to keep driving blindly. Perhaps you'll run across a gas station when you need one. Another option is to look at a map to get a sense of what's ahead. With a map, you can better plan your route. You might even enjoy the ride.

A rising viral load could just be a blip

Say you're tooting along on HIV medicine and everything is going well. Your T-cells are up and your viral load are less than 40 copies. Then, one day your doctor ruins your groove with the news that your viral load is up a bit. There's a chance it's just a viral blip, an intermittent spike of low-level virus. This just happens sometimes in people on successful HIV medicine.

If your viral load had been undetectable (below 40 copies) and then blips, this is not a bad sign according to research. Viral blips are not associated with treatment failure and do not predict failure, at least in drug-naïve people.

A viral blip is a viral load of more than 50 copies in someone who was previously below 50 copies for an extended length of time. It's only a blip if the next viral load test shows the viral levels to be below 50 once again. Two consecutive viral load results above 200 copies is considered to be treatment failure, at least by most doctors. According to Daniel S. Berger, M.D., medical director of Northstar Medical Center in Chicago, "even *two* viral loads above 50 may just be one blip that takes longer to come down."

There was a time when doctors and researchers blamed viral blips entirely on the patient not being adherent. Now, doctors know that blips can happen even if the patient is completely adherent to their meds. Doctors now think that blips may be caused by fluctuating levels of HIV medicine in the blood or that the virus is getting cleaned out from hard-to-reach areas of your body.

A rising viral load over time is not a blip

Don't sweat over a one-time blip in viral load. However, if the blip doesn't go away, it becomes a different ballgame. "If sequential viral load testing shows a trend of increasing viral levels, and they are increasing to concerning levels—say they are 200, then 800, then 1,200, and then 1,500—obviously that's failing. Changing the regimen should be considered," says Dr. Berger.

"But if [one viral load test is] 200 or 300, I wouldn't necessarily say you're failing the regimen, especially if you're feeling well and not having any difficulty in taking the medication." Berger explained that when a viral load begins to climb in a patient, he inquires about the patient's adherence to meds.

"You want to be absolutely sure that you're taking the medications 100 percent of the time, not 80 or 85 percent of the time. That might be the difference," says Dr. Berger. "So you may not be failing the regimen, you may just be failing *taking* the regimen. In which case, if you get back on the wagon and take the medications 100 percent of the time, the viral levels usually come back down."

For better or worse, many people who test positive for HIV these days may not be as motivated as people were in the past. "There's this entire generation of people whose direct involvement with HIV was after the mid-1990s," says Bob Munk, an HIV advocate and operator of the AIDS InfoNet. "They never saw their friends get sick and die. So, they have a skewed risk-benefit assessment internally for anti-viral therapy. They don't really see the benefits with the same clarity that they see the side effects."

Dr. Berger concurs, adding that many people today are younger, in their late teens and early twenties. "They didn't see people during the 1980s and early 1990s walking around the street with their bones showing, looking like skeletons, and often with purple spots on their face, depicting hallmarks of Kaposi's sarcoma, and appearing very sickly," says Dr. Berger. "So they don't have a frame of reference or understand what it means to have AIDS."

Not being adherent isn't always your fault

"So I go get this new job and it's really demanding," says Alan G. "I'm not about to take my meds during a staff meeting. Try timing medicine and food at a Thanksgiving dinner. Imagine landing in Peru for work, while your luggage (and meds) land in Colombia. I'm a fairly organized guy, but I'm no Superman."

On one hand, we all know that treatment adherence is important. On the other hand, we are just human and sometimes we get tired, lazy, or forgetful. "A while back, my doctor asked if I missed doses of medicine. I said 'yes.' He looked disappointed, wrote something in my chart, and then delivered a four-minute speech that left me with anxiety and guilt," says Alan G.

"Now when my doc asks the same question, I think for a moment. 'Do I want the speech or not? I'm sure I miss a dose now and then, but I don't admit to it," he says. "It's just easier."

An acquaintance of mine fibs to his doctor as well. Not only does he miss meds for the usual reasons, but he occasionally takes extended drug and alcohol getaways. He's a party boy and likes circuit parties where it's easy to buy underground drugs such as cocaine, special K, ecstasy, or crystal. He knows it's unwise to mix HIV meds with street drugs, so he opts for the street drugs and lies to his doctor.

But lying to your doctor is also lying to yourself. If you've made the decision to start HIV medicine, but you find yourself telling white lies to your doctor, the problem just might be with your doctor. "Find a physician who you can be very comfortable with, that you can tell everything to, not one that you have to hide things from," advises Dr. Berger.

Research shows that patients treated by doctors with more HIV experience tend to fare a little better. Research also shows that it's unlikely you'll be 100 percent adherent to your meds over the course of years. So it's up to your doctor to match the right drug combination to the right patient.

"See a physician that has experience with HIV, that has been doing this for a long time, not somebody that has a few patients that happen to be HIV-positive," says Dr. Berger. "I try to make it very easy, because if I make it easy for the patient, then he or she is more apt to continue taking or adhere to the medication regimen. By doing so, it will remain effective for a lot longer than not."

"Patients often ask me, how long will this last? They've heard that perhaps 18 months is the average time that these regimens last," he says. "Some studies have been done to see what the average time was on the initial regimen. I wonder about which regimens these patients were initially offered. Were they put on difficult regimens?"

Berger explains that he steers away from offering three-times-a-day regimens or regimens that require an empty stomach four times a day. "I don't know how physicians can actually put a person on such a regimen," he says. "What kind of thought process was involved when a physician puts a patient on a regimen that's difficult to take and potentially has more side effects?"

"Ideally, people should be able to trust their doc," says Munk. "But plenty of people have raised questions about physicians who are intimately involved in researching new products and whether they are sufficiently objective or get swept in the enthusiasm. That's certainly what I'd like to think, that just they're get swept up in the enthusiasm."

The bottom line is that a blip or short-term rise in viral load is probably not a reason for concern. "If patients do remain on the medicine, they can go far beyond what has been shown in some statistically in studies," says Dr. Berger.

IN A SENTENCE:

> *A temporary rise in viral load while on HIV treatment can mean many things.*

learning

Understanding Second-Line HIV Medicine

IF YOUR HIV viral load was below 40 or 50 copies for an extended period, and then it jumps higher on two consecutive occasions, most doctors would agree this to be first-line HIV medicine failure, assuming viral blips or adherence can be ruled out.

At the end of the day, the problem is resistance. If first-line medicine fails, HIV has become resistant to one or all of the drugs in your combination. Think of the virus as a forest fire and your three-drug combo as three different fire roads. For whatever reason, the fire jumped at least one of the roads and is now burning away on the other side.

Keep in mind that once you've taken HIV medicine, you lose the title *drug-naïve*. Your new category: *treatment experienced*. If you've ever taken HIV medicine, you're considered treatment experienced. Goals for those with extensive treatment experience can differ somewhat from those who are drug naïve.

One man's failure is another man's success

HIV medicine changes fast, according to Daniel S. Berger, M.D., medical director of Northstar Medical. "It continues to shift with every passing year. HIV treatment is continuing to evolve, not from decade to decade—but month to month and week to week."

For example, today's definition of *treatment failure* is very different from what it was a few years ago. At one time, treatment failure meant an AIDS-defining opportunistic infection. Today, it means two consecutive viral loads above 50 copies or T-cells below a specific threshold, say 200.

To put it another way, *treatment failure* is really just an artificial milestone, agreed upon by you and your doctor. Some people can negotiate with their doctors to agree on what constitutes treatment failure, says Bob Munk. "Say you're a person who would get freaked out about sunken cheeks, then have an agreement with your doc, that 'we'll try this regimen until I start seeing signs of sunken cheeks, then we're going to switch to something else.'"

Expectations for second-line treatment are different

Your expectation should be a little less for a second-line treatment compared to a first-line regimen. If you're treatment experienced or have resistance, you will find that remaining HIV drugs are far less convenient to take and may cause more side effects.

"We try to reduce the propensity of side effects, reduce the potential for the development of metabolic problems and lipodystrophy while reducing the risks for other long-term complications," says Dr. Berger.

So the goals for the drug-naïve patient and treatment-experienced patient are somewhat different.

Treatment interruptions between regimens are dicey

If your first-line HIV medicine has failed, you might consider taking a temporary break from all anti-HIV drugs. Treatment interruptions are being studied in a range of settings, however, but the research does not show a benefit.

What's clear, at this point, is that treatment interruptions can cause significant decreases of T-cells and increases in viral load.

"I think that's something that hasn't been completely worked out yet," says Dr. Berger. "We don't know how often or how long a treatment interruption should occur. We don't know all the strategies that are possible. We do know that a lot of factors can contribute to [treatment] failure.

"Not only is [the problem] resistant mutations, but sometimes it's poor or lower drug absorption, maybe the presence of compartments where drugs can't get into to achieve the appropriate levels needed to suppress the virus," says Dr. Berger. "If those are the problems, then going off treatment won't solve that part of the problem."

Resistance testing helps you make better choices about drugs

You don't really need to know exactly *how* resistance tests work, in order to understand what it means. There are two types of tests: **genotypic** and **phenotypic.**

Genotypic tests use a sample of your blood to identify mutations in the virus that are resistant to specific drugs. Genotypic tests use DNA, special chemicals, and computers to produce a snapshot of the virus that's inside you and only you. The snapshot is a picture of the "resistance mutations" that your virus has created to survive.

These mutations are given names, such as "M41" or "184V." For example, if you have an M41 mutation it might mean that Drug A will no longer work for you. On the other hand, if you have a 184V mutation, it might mean that both Drug A and Drug B won't work. Interpreting mutations is complicated and getting more so every day.

Phenotype tests use a sample of your blood. But this time, HIV is grown in your laboratory sample and it's then tested against different HIV drugs to see what works and what doesn't.

"I think genotypic testing is too limited," notes Dr. Berger. "A genotypic test gives you the mutations that can be isolated from a particular patient, but if the physician doesn't completely understand how to interpret the results, they can easily be misinterpreted. The physician may be falsely interpreting [the results], when, in fact, the patient does have a lot of options."

A recent study of health-care professionals caring for people with HIV found that only about a quarter of them can accurately match the majority of genotypic HIV resistance mutations to the drug class affected. Guidelines exist to recommend the use of genotypic testing for HIV patients, but proper interpretation of the results is harder to come by.

The International AIDS Society–USA provides doctors with a resistance mutation chart for interpreting genotyping results (online at http://www.iasusa.org). The chart is continuously updated and provides user notes to explain the significance of specific mutations.

Virlogic does have a test called a PhenoSense GT, which combines the two tests," says Berger. "They also provide for free a lab test called a viral "'replicative capacity.' When HIV becomes resistant to some drugs, it also

CONSTRUCTING A SECOND-LINE TREATMENT IN THE EVENT THAT FIRST-LINE TREATMENT FAILS:

	Drug 1	Drug 2	Drug 3
PI			
Nuke		tenofovir	emtricitabine
Non-nuke	efavirenz		

SECOND-LINE TREATMENT MIGHT BE:

	Drug 1	Drug 2	Drug 3
PI	atazanavir		
Nuke		didanosine	stavudine
Non-nuke			

loses some of its strength or 'fitness.' In other words, although viral loads persist in the blood, a reduced replicative capacity indicates that the virus is crippled and has a reduced ability to kill T-cells." Research has shown that measuring viral fitness can provide valuable information that can guide you and your healthcare provider in making better treatment decisions. "In other words, even if there's resistance—if the [viral fitness] is low—you're more likely to maintain immune function."

Second-line treatment is a second chance to control the virus

"It's like a chess game. You always have to think a couple of moves in advance," says Dr. Berger. "Treatments are limited, but there's going be a move, a move after that, and a move after that. Our treatment approach has evolved in this way out of necessity, ensuring that patients have as many later options as possible."

Dr. Berger explains that certain medicines have the potential for causing other medications to be ruled out in the future. In other words, using Drug A can rule out using Drug B at a later time. This sequence, he says, has to be carefully considered.

Optimism among the HIV community has come with the introduction of newer classes of drugs, such as the fusion inhibitors, including Fuzeon (enfuvirtide). However, the optimism is primary for **salvage therapy**, which is a last-ditch—but potent—attempt to snuff out the virus.

"I'm very forthright and honest with patients that if they wanted to explore [Fuzeon], it's open," says Dr. Berger. "But they need to understand that the drug is self-injected twice daily and it's very expensive. For people who are at a later stage and have exhausted options, it's a very important drug and should not be overlooked. It can be a lifesaving drug, but it has its limitations. The landscape of HIV medicine is a dynamic entity with continuous evolution and change. Therefore, patients can be more hopeful about the future."

IN A SENTENCE:

> If first-line HIV medicine fails, physician experience and resistance testing can help guide choices for second-time medicine.

You Can Have Children

BECAUSE YOU'RE human, you were built to survive. This survival instinct is weaved into your DNA, cells, emotions, and your everyday behavior. But when there's no immediate threat to your well-being, you, like all humans, start looking around for something more.

Eventually, you'll understand that HIV is no longer a threat to you. Your planning, healthy behaviors, medical care, treatment strategies, adherence to medicine will all come together and tip the scales toward feeling safe and assured about your future. You'll start to feel like a regular human being again.

There was a time when having HIV meant *not* having children. Doctors and health officials generally agreed that people with HIV wouldn't live long enough to care for children. That was when—for HIV-positive women—the high risk of passing the virus to the baby during delivery was unacceptable. For HIV-positive men, the central issue was the unacceptable risk of passing the virus to the mother.

. . .

Those obstacles have been overcome. Those days are gone. And don't let anybody tell you otherwise. The right to procreate is central to personal identity, dignity, and to the meaning of one's life.

Now, whether you actually want children is a different matter. That decision is up to you. Just know that if you decide that you do want children, it *is* possible.

Here's a look at why this consensus has changed over the years, a few considerations to keep in mind, and some specific suggestions on how to make it all happen—for both women and for men.

Women with HIV can safely have healthy children

"If a woman wants to have children, she can. HIV is not going to stop her from having children," says Precious J., of Women Alive, an AIDS service organization in Los Angeles, California. "Thank God, we do have medication that can reduce the transmission of HIV to the baby."

Years ago, before effective medicine for HIV, the risk of a woman passing the virus to her child during pregnancy was as high as 30 percent. Today, through the judicious use of HIV medicine, delivery by cesarean section, and avoidance of breast-feeding, this risk is now less than 2 percent—a risk to the baby that's comparable to HIV-negative women over the age of 40, or those with diabetes.

Recent studies also show that HIV-positive women who get pregnant do not get any sicker than those who are not pregnant. That is, becoming pregnant does not appear to be dangerous to the health of an HIV-positive woman.

Potential harmful effects to the baby by HIV medicine—taken by the mother during pregnancy—remain a concern. For many years, it was common for pregnant women to take zidovudine (Retrovir) alone. However, a recent study of women with HIV who gave birth showed a dramatic change in the individual medications taken by women during pregnancy.

The study showed that the use of zidovudine decreased from 96 percent during the early 1990s to only 6 percent during 2001. During the same time, use of three-drug regimens that included a protease inhibitor increased to 41 percent, and regimens that included a non-nucleoside reverse transcriptase inhibitors (non-nuke) increased to 43 percent.

Researchers have studied the use of HIV medicine during the first, second, and third trimesters of pregnancy and observed no increase in birth defects. They concluded that, while the results are preliminary, this research does provide "some reassurance" regarding the trends of using three-drug combinations during pregnancy.

However, they also cautioned that there's not enough long-term research about the risks of some specific drugs. Either way, the research is helpful in discussing options for women taking HIV medicine who are considering pregnancy. It should be noted that efavirenz (Sustiva) has been shown to cause birth defects in animals.

Some doctors are rethinking the generally supported view that the use of a cesarean ("C") section to reduce the possibility of transmitting the virus from mother to child during labor. In a presentation at a recent AIDS conference, Karen P. Beckerman, M.D., director of the Bay Area Perinatal AIDS Center at the University of California, San Francisco, suggested that there's not enough evidence to support the notion that healthy HIV-infected pregnant women should routinely be offered C-sections. Clearly, more research is needed.

Can women with HIV create a family? "Yes, and I've seen it," says Jelka Jonker, a counselor and therapist at AIDS Project Los Angeles. However, she said that women should first go through all the stages of emotions that come with a new diagnosis of HIV. They need to become comfortable themselves first.

There are going to be obstacles. According to Jonker, HIV-positive women have a harder time finding a partner. "Say a woman finds somebody and they decide to have children, a lot of people are going to be very judgmental. Some people think 'How can you be so selfish?' Or, 'You might not live that long.' So it's not easy. You have to be a really strong person to overcome all of that."

Men want children—whether they verbalize it or not

Straight or gay, almost every man values the idea of having offspring, whether he verbalizes it or not. Men are imbedded with the desire to procreate. Men who seek the same gender for sexual expression are still following the same natural human instincts for procreation as those who prefer the opposite gender.

"The very first thought I had when I tested positive was that I'd never have kids," says Mark H. "I don't know why, but that part bothered me the most."

With new technology, HIV-positive men can father children without passing on the virus. Fertility researchers have developed a technique called "sperm washing" where sperm is isolated from fluid and white blood

HIV

cells—the place most likely for HIV to hide. If doctors don't find HIV in the sperm sample, then it is joined with an egg through *in vitro* fertilization.

In vitro fertilization is a process that involves retrieving eggs from ovaries, placing them in special solutions, and combining the sperm and eggs in a dish. The resulting embryos are placed in an incubator where they're nourished until maturity. At the appropriate time, the pre-embryos are removed from the dish and replaced in the uterus, where they continue on with normal fetal development.

Only a handful of fertility centers in the United States have experience with these techniques, which have given life to many healthy, HIV-negative children as well as protected their mothers from the virus. Ideal candidates are men with low or undetectable levels of HIV.

Help with fertility is there if you want it

The American Society for Reproductive Medicine (ASRM) now offers guidelines for treating infertility in people with HIV. The guidelines examine several different scenarios and issues. The document offers information for different situations, such as when only one partner has HIV or when both partners have HIV.

According to the ASRM, doctors who practice reproductive medicine should not deny treatment to individuals with HIV. Ethically and legally, fertility doctors have the same obligation to treat patients with HIV as they do patients with any other chronic illness. When a clinic lacks the skills and facilities to manage people with HIV, the clinic should provide a referral to another clinic that has these resources.

"With the development of new techniques and treatment protocols, we're able now to help HIV-positive patients have children while minimizing the risks they face," says William Keye, Jr., M.D., president of the American Society of Reproductive Medicine.

"A lot of times in our society, we always say what people should do—until we are in that position—and then we should do something different," says Rosetta M., who also works in the health education field. However, she adds, generally people in the United States don't take advantage of adoption or becoming a foster parent. Still, she contends that people with HIV should have the right to procreate.

"HIV is like any other disease or genetic condition, you don't know what the future holds," says Rosetta M. If people with HIV "should not" have kids, she argues, then if you work two jobs and can't stay home, you shouldn't have kids either. If you have herpes, you shouldn't have kids. If you have substance abuse in your family, you shouldn't have kids. Where do we stop?"

For more information on pregnancy and HIV

American Society for Reproductive Medicine
1209 Montgomery Highway
Birmingham, Alabama 35216
(205) 978-5000

Jones Institute for Reproductive Medicine
601 Colley Ave
Norfolk, VA 23507
(800) 515-6637

IN A SENTENCE:

> *If you have HIV, it is possible to safely have healthy children.*

learning

Keep Moving Forward

SO WHAT does the future look like for HIV? It's hard to say. Finding a cure for HIV may be possible in our lifetime. After all, there were no effective treatments before 1996, and now there are many. In looking forward, it's hard to predict what might happen. Conventional wisdom may suddenly shift. More research will become available with time. New drugs, better combinations, novel blood tests, and vaccines will be invented. HIV medicine is an evolving science.

New and better drugs coming down the pipeline is good reason for optimism, according to Anthony Fauci, M.D., director of the National Institute of Allergy and Infectious Diseases. He notes that over the next few years, new HIV drugs will be developed that specifically target HIV in different ways than the older drugs.

The future of HIV medicine, Fauci says, will "skirt away from the protease reverse transcriptase inhibitors and common [cross resistant] prototype drugs. It's a work in progress—that's the good news and the bad news. It's not absolute now."

So how do you keep track of HIV medicine as it changes over time? First, decide if it's even worth your time. Everyone is different. Some people choose only to learn about HIV medicine as they need it, so they can get on with the business of living. Other people monitor newsletters and Web sites on occasion. A few get more involved by "giving back" or volunteering.

Giving back can mean many things

"I don't think there's an obligation to give back," says Rosetta M., who also works in the health education field. "First, figure out where you are emotionally, before you try to branch out and give away pieces of yourself. I think there are other ways people can give back, by living healthy—living a prosperous life—and I don't mean financial.

"Being happy, that's giving back," says Rosetta M. "Then there's one less miserable bitch walking around. Just being able to walk outside and say hi to somebody else—'good morning' and smile or whatever—you're giving back."

With time, some people with HIV get involved in things that are meaningful for them. "If you know that you've been helped and you've gone through all those emotions—and if you came out as a better person—helping others can change your attitude toward life," says Jelke Jonker, a counselor at AIDS Project Los Angeles.

"People have told me that being HIV-positive has changed their life in a better way because they now have a more productive attitude toward life. Obviously, that's not true for everybody. But a lot of people have told me that."

Some people are driven by civic or moral duty so they turn outward and gain satisfaction from helping others. Other people are driven more out of self-interest and ask, "What's in it for me?" Humans are complicated beings; we're both selfless and selfish at the same time.

If you've had some good fortune along the way, if somebody took you under their wing at some point, then I think you owe a little something. Think of it as "fee for services" if that suits you better.

So how do you pay it forward? One way is to volunteer at an AIDS service organization, or become a facilitator for people who are newly diagnosed, or just be nice to other people. "What better way to give back for the things you have received when you needed them?" says Jonker.

Keeping up with the details of HIV can't hurt

Most people with HIV get their medical news from their doctor, newsletters, or the Internet. In all three cases, you might not be able to judge the quality of the information you are getting from these sources. One way is to diversify your sources of information. For example, you might learn something in a newsletter and then ask your doctor for his thoughts on the same subject. Here's a look at some reliable and trustworthy sources of information:

If activism inspires you

WANT TO do something but you don't know how to start? Here's a short list of key organizations involved with HIV politics and policy.

AIDS ACTION

AIDS Action is a political group that keeps tabs on national policies regarding HIV. In a sense, the group educates and "motivates" elected officials so that people with HIV are represented on a national level.

AIDS Action
1703 M Street NW, Suite 611
Washington, DC 20036
(202) 530-8030
http://www.aidsaction.org

SURVIVE AIDS

Survive AIDS is the new name for what was once called ACT UP Golden Gate. It is a grassroots, all-volunteer group of individuals in San Francisco, California, who work in different ways to ensure adequate funding and resources for the care, treatment, and prevention of HIV.

Survive AIDS
584 Castro Street, PMB 542
San Francisco, CA 94114
(415) 252-9200
http://www.surviveaids.org

ACT UP NEW YORK

ACT UP is a diverse, non-partisan group of individuals committed to direct action to end the AIDS crisis. The group's motto: "Our job is not to be invited to coffee or to schmooze at a cocktail party. Our job is to make change happen as fast as possible and direct action works for that." The group meets every Monday at 8:00 p.m.

ACT UP/New York
208 W. 13th Street
New York, NY 10011
(212) 630-7310
http://www.actupny.org

POZ MAGAZINE

Poz is a four-color glossy magazine published in New York City. *Poz* is engaging, accessible, and isn't homework. It's very conversational, pleasing to look at, and tuned into culture and lifestyle issues. The magazine is free to people who cannot afford a subscription—one year of twelve issues is $19.97. (It's well worth the money.) Make sure you specifically request that the company doesn't make your name available to other groups.

Poz magazine
500 Fifth Avenue, Suite 320
New York, NY 10110
(212) 242-2163
http://www.poz.com

POSITIVELY AWARE

Positively Aware is magazine-like in that it's printed in four-color, but it feels and reads more like a "grassroots," treatment-focused publication. Given the technical nature of HIV treatment, *Positively Aware* offers a respectable choice of plain-language articles and commentary. The publication produces an annual "drug guide" that is particularly noteworthy.

Positively Aware
Test Positive Aware Network
5537 N. Broadway Street
Chicago, IL 60640
(773) 989-9400
http://www.tpan.com

AIDS INFONET.ORG

AIDS InfoNet is a Web site originally designed to make information on HIV services and treatments easily accessible in English and Spanish for residents of New Mexico. However, the Web site has become widely acclaimed for its non-technical fact sheets, which are updated frequently to reflect advances in medicine, and are available in both English and Spanish.

New Mexico AIDS InfoNet
PO Box 810
Arroyo Seco, NM 87514
http://www.aidsinfonet.org

HIVandHepatitis.com

HIVandHepatitis.com is a Web site based in San Francisco, California. It offers a steady stream of accurate, timely, and cutting-edge information about treatment for HIV, hepatitis B, and hepatitis C. It's especially unique in that issues related to co-infections are well covered.

HIVandHepatitis.com
PO Box 14288
San Francisco, CA 94114
http://www.hivandhepatitis.com

Natap.org

NATAP is a New York-based non-profit organization that operates a no-nonsense Web site focused primarily on HIV and hepatitis C treatment. The Web site offers the latest developments in treatment with a clear commitment to objectivity and deciphering fact from the claims of the pharmaceutical companies.

NATAP
580 Broadway, Suite 1010
New York, NY 10012
(212) 219-0106
http://www.natap.org

You are now armed for life

You now are armed with the knowledge and the tools you need to survive HIV. You have an understanding of the virus, your own emotions, getting proper medical care, sexually transmitted diseases, mental health, nutrition, exercise, strategies for HIV medicine, and a dose of hope for the future. The choice to act on this knowledge is now your own. Like it or not, you're in control. You can make smart choices over time. Or not. Better choices over time spin the odds in your favor. The choice is yours.

IN A SENTENCE:

> *Giving back and staying connected to HIV organizations, newsletters, and Web sites can help you make better choices in the future.*

Glossary

ACUTE INFECTION: The phase of HIV infection when the blood contains many viral particles that spread throughout the body, seeding themselves in various organs, particularly the lymphoid tissues.

AIDS COCKTAIL: Another name for **combination therapy.**

AMPHETAMINE: Drugs that speed up the way your body works. They make your heart work faster, and they pump adrenaline into the system. The user feels more energetic, cheerful, and confident, and because of these effects there is a high risk of psychological dependence.

ANGIOTENSIN CONVERTING ENZYME (ACE) INHIBITORS: Medications that lower blood pressure and are commonly prescribed for the treatment of high blood pressure (hypertension).

ANILINGUS: Erotic stimulation achieved by contact between mouth and anus.

ANTIRETROVIRALS: Drugs that work by interfering with the HIV life cycle. When used in combination, these medications reduce the amount of virus in the blood and help to delay the progress of disease.

ANTIVIRALS: Drugs that work by changing the genetic material of the host cell so that the virus cannot use the host's genetic material as efficiently.

ANXIETY: An emotional state in which people feel uneasy, apprehensive, or fearful.

ASPARTATE TRANSAMINASE (AST): A type of enzyme that is found in blood serum and certain body tissues, especially the heart and the liver.

ASPERGILLOSIS: An infection with, or disease caused by, molds.

ASYMPTOMATIC SHEDDING: Occurs when the herpes virus is released in genital secretions or on the skin when the sores or lesions that mark an active genital herpes outbreak are absent, and is a major vehicle of transmission of the genital herpes virus.

BAREBACKING: Generally refers to gay men engaging in unprotected anal intercourse.

BENZODIAZEPINE: A class of commonly prescribed tranquilizers that can cause addiction.

bDNA (BRANCHED DNA): A test that combines a material that gives off light with the sample. This material connects with the HIV particles. The amount of light is measured and converted to a viral count.

BUSPIRONE (BuSPAR): A medication that relieves anxiety with minimal sedation, minimal muscle relaxation, and no addiction potential.

CANDIDIASIS (THRUSH, YEAST INFECTION): A fungal infection characterized by white patches in the mouth, difficulty swallowing, and, in women, vaginal irritation and thick, white discharge.

CD4 CELL: One of the two main types of T-cells, also known as helper cells, which leads the attack against infections.

COMBINATION THERAPY: Using more than one drug at a time.

CUNNILINGUS: Oral stimulation of the vulva or clitoris.

DENTAL DAM: A small sheet of latex which acts as a barrier between the vagina or anus and the mouth.

DIABETES MELLITUS: A condition characterized by raised concentration of sugar in the blood and urine, due to problems with the production or action of insulin.

DIACETYLMORPHINE: A highly addictive morphine derivative.

DISASSOCIATION: The separation of whole segments of the personality (as in multiple personality) or of discrete mental processes (as in the schizophrenia) from the mainstream of consciousness or of behavior.

DNA: Deoxyribonucleic acid, the material in the nucleus of a cell where genetic information is stored.

DYSPLASIA: An abnormal growth or development of organs or cells.

ECSTASY: A synthetic amphetamine analogue used illicitly for its mood-enhancing and hallucinogenic properties.

EPISODIC THERAPY: Taking medication only during an outbreak to speed healing.

GENOTYPIC: A type of drug resistance testing that directly exposes a person's virus to antiviral drugs to determine how much of the drug is required to block viral activity.

GLUCOSE: A form of sugar found in the bloodstream. All sugars and starches are converted into glucose before they are absorbed.

HEPATITIS C VIRUS (HVC): A form of liver inflammation that causes rapidly developing and often chronic disease.

HIGHLY ACTIVE ANTIRETROVIRAL THERAPY (HAART): A term used to describe anti-HIV combination therapy with three or more drugs.

HUMAN PAPILLOMA VIRUS (HPV): A group of wart-causing viruses which are also responsible for cancer of the cervix and some anal cancers.

HYPOCHONDRIA: Extreme depression of the mind and spirit often centered on imaginary physical ailments.

KAPOSI'S SARCOMA: A cancer characterized by red or purple blotches on the skin or mucous membranes; may also affect internal organs.

LIPODYSTROPHY: A disruption to the way the body produces, uses, and distributes fat among people taking anti-HIV therapy.

LIPOHYPERTROPHY: Abnormal fat gains that usually occur around the gut, waist, and back of the neck.

LOG: Short for logarithm, a scale of measurement often used when describing viral load. A one-log change is a tenfold change, such as from 100 to 10. A two-log change is a hundredfold change, such as from 1,000 to 10.

METHAMPHETAMINE: A drug that works directly on the brain and spinal cord by interfering with normal neurotransmission. Neurotransmitters are chemical substances naturally produced within nerve cells used to communicate with each other and send messages to influence and regulate our thinking and all other systems throughout the body.

METHYLENEDIOXYMETHAMPHETAMINE (MDMA): See **ecstasy.**

MONOAMINE OXIDASE INHIBITORS (MAOIs): Medicines that relieve certain types of mental depression.

NONOXYNOL-9: A spermicide used in contraceptive products.

OPPORTUNISTIC INFECTIONS: Specific infections that cause disease in someone with a damaged immune system.

PARTIAL SEROTONIN REUPTAKE INHIBITORS: A group of chemically unique antidepressant drugs that are effective in depression, bulimia nervosa, obsessive compulsive disorder, anorexia nervosa, panic disorder, pain associated with diabetic neuropathy, and for premenstrual syndrome.

PATHOGENESIS: The origination and development of a disease.

PHENOTYPIC: A type of drug resistance testing that measures the amount of drug needed to suppress the growth of HIV in a laboratory setting.

PILL BURDEN: The number of pills you're required to take each day as part of your HIV drug therapy.

PNEUMOCYSTIS CARINII PNEUMONIA (PCP): A parasite that infects the lungs, causing fever, dry cough, shortness of breath. PCP is an AIDS-defining illness.

PCR (POLYMERASE CHAIN REACTION): A test that uses an enzyme to multiply the HIV in the blood sample. Then a chemical reaction marks the virus. The markers are measured and used to calculate the amount of virus.

PRODROME: A symptom of disease that warns you of its presence.

PROTEASE INHIBITOR (PI): Family of antiretrovirals that target the protease enzyme. Includes amprenavir, indinavir, lopinavir, ritonavir, saquinavir, nelfinavir, and atazanavir.

PSYCHOTHERAPY: Treatment of mental or emotional disorder or of related bodily ills by psychological means.

QI: An Eastern medicine term for the body's flow of energy.

RETROVIRUS: Family of viruses to which HIV belongs, that are distinguished by their use of RNA.

RNA: Ribonucleic acid, the form in which HIV stores its genetic material.

SALVAGE THERAPY: A course of action for people who have become fully or partially resistant to current drugs and are seeking drugs in new classes, older drugs to recycle, and other treatment strategies that may slow HIV and make their bodies' immune systems run efficiently again.

SEDATIVE: An agent or a drug having a soothing, calming, or tranquilizing effect.

SEROTONIN: A neurotransmitter involved in many behaviors, including human mood disorders and aggressive behaviors.

SEXUALLY TRANSMITTED DISEASE (STD): Any of various diseases transmitted by direct sexual contact that include venereal diseases (as syphilis, gonorrhea, and chancroid) and other diseases (as hepatitis A, hepatitis B, giardiasis, and AIDS) that are often or sometimes contracted by other than sexual means.

SURROGATE MARKERS: An indirect indicater of something, such as measuring viral load to assess the treatment effect of a drug.

SUPPRESSIVE THERAPY: Taking an antiviral medication daily as a preventative measure, to keep HSV in check, reduce flare-ups, and lessen symptoms.

T-CELLS: A type of lymphocyte (white blood cell) that constitutes an important part of the immune system.

TETRAHYDROCANNABINOL (THC): A physiologically active chemical from hemp plant resin that is the chief intoxicant in marijuana.

TRICYCLICS: Antidepressants that relieve mental depression.

VIRAL LOAD: The amount of HIV virus in the blood.

Bibliography

Day 1: Living

1. Hogg, R., et al. "Improved Survival Among HIV-infected Individuals Following Initiation of Antiretroviral Therapy." *Journal of the American Medical Association* 1998; 279: 450–454.
2. Palella, F., et al. "Declining Morbidity and Mortality Among Patients with Advanced Human Immunodeficiency Virus Infection." *New England Journal of Medicine* 1998; 338: 853–860.
3. Smith, R. (Editor). *Encyclopedia of AIDS: A Social, Political, Cultural, and Scientific Record of the HIV Epidemic*, (New York: Penguin, 2001).

Day 1: Learning

1. The Henry J. Kaiser Family Foundation, HIV/AIDS Policy Fact Sheet. November www.kff.org. 2006.
2. Center for Disease Control. "Revised Recommendations for HIV Testing of Adults, Adolescents, and Pregnant Women in Health-Care Settings." *Morbidity and Mortality Weekly Report (MMWR)*, 55(RR14);1–17. September 22, 2006.
3. *HIV/AIDS Surveillance Report: Cases of HIV infection and AIDS in the United States and Dependent Areas*. U.S. Department of Health and Human Services and the Centers for Disease Control and Prevention (CDC). Vol. 17. 2005.

Day 2: Living

1. Samet, J., et al. "Trillion Virion Delay: Time from Testing Positive for HIV to Presentation for Primary Care." *Archives of Internal Medicine* 1998; 158: 734–40.
2. Leserman, J., et al. "Impact of stressful life events, depression, social support, coping, and cortisol on progression to AIDS." *American Journal of Psychiatry* 2000 Aug; 157(8):1221–8.
3. Canadian Psychiatric Association, *HIV & Psychiatry: A Training and Resource Manual*. Ottawa, Ontario: 2000.
4. Power, R., et al. "Self-disclosure of HIV serostatus in relation to depression and social support." Abstract. XIV International AIDS Conference, Barcelona, Spain, 2002.

Day 2: Learning

1. Collins R., D. Kanouse, A. Gifford, J. Senterfitt, M. Schuster, D. McCaffrey, M. Shapiro, N. Wenger, *Health Psychol.* September;20(5):351–60. 2001.

Day 3: Living

1. Center for Disease Control. "Revised Recommendations for HIV Testing of Adults, Adolescents, and Pregnant Women in Health-Care Settings." *Morbidity and Mortality Weekly Report (MMWR)*, 55(RR14):1–17. September 22, 2006.
2. HIV/AIDS Surveillance Report: Cases of HIV infection and AIDS in the United States and Dependent Areas. U.S. Department of Health and Human Services and the Centers for Disease Control and Prevention. Vol. 17. 2005.

Day 3: Learning

1. Sackoff, J. E., D. B. Hanna, M. R. Pfeiffer, and others. "Causes of death among persons with AIDS in the era of highly active antiretroviral therapy: New York City." *Annals of Internal Medicine* 145(6): 397–406. September 19, 2006.
2. Fauci, Anthony. Personal interview. 2002.
3. Amen, Daniel G. *Making a Good Brain Great: The Amen Clinic Program for Achieving and Sustaining Optimal Mental Performance*, (New York: Three Rivers Press: 2005).
4. Aberg, J. A . "The changing face of HIV care: Common things really are common." *Annals of Internal Medicine* 145(6): 463–465. September 19, 2006.

Day 4: Living

1. Herek, G., J. Capitanio, J., K. Widaman. "HIV-related stigma and knowledge in the United States: Prevalence and trends, 1991–1999." *American Journal of Public Health* 2002 March; 92(3):371–7.

Day 4: Learning

1. Harold, K. "An 83-Year-Old Woman with Chronic Illness and Strong Religious Beliefs." *Journal of the American Medical Association* 2002; 288:487–493.
2. Ironson, G., et al. "The Ironson-Woods Spirituality/Religiousness Index is associated with long survival, health behaviors, less distress, and low cortisol in people with HIV/AIDS. *Ann Behav Med* 2002 Winter; 24(1):34–48.
3. Melbourne, K. "The Impact of Religion on Adherence with Antiretrovirals." *Journal of the Association of Nurses in AIDS Care* (05/99–06/99) Vol. 10, No. 3: 99.
4. "Risks for HIV Infection Among Persons Residing in Rural Areas and Small Cities—Selected Sites, Southern United States, 1995–1996." *Morbidity and Mortality Weekly Report* (11/20/98) Vol. 47, No. 45: 974.

Day 5: Learning

1. Centers for Disease Control & Prevention, "How long does it take for HIV to cause AIDS?" Fact Sheet. November 1998.
2. Centers for Disease Control & Prevention, "How can I tell if I'm infected with HIV? What are the symptoms?" Fact Sheet. November, 1998.
3. F. Hecht, M. Busch, B. Rawal, et al. "Use of laboratory tests and clinical symptoms for identification of primary HIV infection," AIDS 2002, 16:1119–129.
4. R. Weber, L. Christen, M. Loy, S. Schaller, S. Christen, C. Joyce, U. Ledermann, B. Ledergerber, R. Cone, R. Luthy, M.R. Cohen, "Randomized, placebo-controlled trial of Chinese herb therapy for HIV-1-infected individuals," *Journal of Acquired Immune Deficiency Syndrome* 1999 September 1;22(1):56–64.
5. Burack J. M. Cohen, J. Hahn, D. Abrams, "Pilot randomized controlled trial of Chinese herbal treatment for HIV-associated symptoms," *ournal of Acquired Immune Deficiency Syndrome Hum Retrovirol* 1996 August 1;12(4):386–93.
6. Lin X., L. Xu, Y. Feng, J. Li, L. Pei, T. Shen, Y. Shao, "Clinical study on treatment of HIV infected persons based on viral load detection and CD4+T lymphocyte counting," *Zhonghua Shi Yan He Lin Chuang Bing Du Xue Za Zhi.* 2002 Sep;16 (3):211–4.
7. Smith, Raymond A., (Editor), *Encyclopedia of AIDS: A Social, Political, Cultural, and Scientific Record of the HIV Epidemic*, (New York: Penguin, 2001).
8. Centers for Disease Control & Prevention, "Preventing Infections From Pets: A Guide For People with HIV Infection," Fact Sheet. June 1999.
9. Gao F., E. Bailes, D. Robertson, Y. Chen, C. Rodenburg, S. Michael, L. Cummins, L. Arthur, M. Peeters, G. Shaw, P. Sharp, B. Hahn, "Origin of HIV-1 in the chimpanzee Pan troglodytes troglodytes," *Nature* 397, 436–41 (1999).
10. Weis R., R. W. Wrangham, "From Pan to Pandemic," *Nature* 397, 385–6 (1999).
11. Zhu T, Korber B, Nahinias A, et al., "An African HIV-1 Sequence from 1959 and Implications for the Origin of the Epidemic," Nature (02/05/98) Vol. 391, No. 6667: 594.
12. Centers for Disease Control & Prevention, "Questions and Answers: HIV is the Cause of AIDS," Fact Sheet. February, 2001.
13. Centers for Disease Control & Prevention, "How is HIV passed from one person to another?" Fact Sheet. November, 1998.

14. Safren, Steven A., Adam S. Radomsky, Michael W. Otto, and Elizabeth Salomon, "Predictors of Psychological Well-Being in a Diverse Sample of HIV-Positive Patients Receiving Highly Active Antiretroviral Therapy," *Psychosomatics,* 2002; 43: 478–85.
15. Smith, Raymond A. (Editor), *Encyclopedia of AIDS: A Social, Political, Cultural, and Scientific Record of the HIV Epidemic,* (New York: Penguin, 2001).

Day 6: *Living*

1. Kelly, J., et al. "Outcome of cognitive-behavioral and support group brief therapies for depressed, HIV-infected persons." *American Journal of Psychiatry* 1993 November; 150(11):1679–86.
2. Kelly, J., et al. "Factors associated with severity of depression and high-risk sexual behavior among persons diagnosed with human immunodeficiency virus (HIV) infection." *Journal of Health Psychology* 1993 May; 12(3):215–9.

Day 6: *Learning*

1. Normand, J., D. Vlahov, L. Moses, (eds.). *Preventing HIV Transmission: The Role of Sterile Needles and Bleach,* (Washington, DC: National Academy Press, 1995).
2. Centers for Disease Control & Prevention. "Update: Syringe Exchange Programs—United States." *Morbidity and Mortality Weekly Report* 1998; 47:652–5.
3. Hagan, H., et al. "Volunteer bias in nonrandomized evaluations of the efficacy of needle-exchange programs." *Journal of Urban Health* 2000; 77:103–12.
4. Groseclose, S., et al. "Impact of increased legal access to needles and syringes on the practices of injecting-drug users and police officers—Connecticut, 1992–93." *Journal of Acquired Immune Deficiency Syndromes and Human Retrovirology* 1995; 10:82–9.
5. Academy for Educational Development. "Comprehensive approach: preventing bloodborne infections among injection drug users." Washington, DC: Academy for Educational Development, 2000. Available at http://www.cdc.gov/idu.

Day 7: *Learning*

1. Mellors, J., A. Munoz, J. Giorgi, J. Margolick, C. Tassoni, P. Gupta, L. Kingsley, J. Todd, A. Saah, R. Detels, J. Phair, C. Rinaldo, "Plasma viral load and CD4+ lymphocytes as prognostic markers of HIV-1 infection," *Ann Internal Medicine.* 1997 June 15;126(12):946–54. (also be found as Table V on page 39 of the August 13, 2001 issue of the "Guidelines for the Use of Antiretroviral Agents in HIV-infected Adults and Adolescents").
2. Samet, J., K. Freedberg, M. Stein, R. Lewis, J. Savetsky, L. Sullivan, S. Levenson, R. Hingson, "Trillion Virion Delay: Time From Testing Positive for HIV to Presentation for Primary Care," *Arch Internal Medicine.* 1998;158:734–40.
3. Leserman J, Petitto J, Golden R, et al. "Impact of stressful life events, depression, social support, coping, and cortisol on progression to AIDS," *American Journal Psychiatry* 2000 August;157(8):1221–8.
4. Canadian Psychiatric Association, *HIV & Psychiatry: A Training and Resource Manual.* (Ottawa, Ontario: 2000).

5. Power, R., L. Duran, Palmer, C. Koopman, C. Gore-Felton, D. Israelski, J. Porter, D. Spiegel, "Self-disclosure of HIV serostatus in relation to depression and social support," Abstract. XIV International AIDS Conference, Barcelona, Spain, 2002.

Week 2: Living

1. Kitahata, M., et al. "Physicians' Experience with the Acquired Immunodeficiency Syndrome as a Factor in Patients' Survival." *New England Journal of Medicine*, Vol. 334:701–07 March 14, 1996, Number 11.
2. More, P., "Is Your Doctor in Financial Trouble?" *Thrive Magazine*, AIDS Health-care Foundation. 2001.
3. Jecker, N., C. Braddock, "Managed Care." *Ethics in Medicine* 1998. University of Washington School of Medicine.
4. Herrick, D. "Would National Health Insurance Benefit Physicians?" Brief Analysis. No. 370, August 31, 2001, National Center for Policy Analysis.
5. Mechanic, D., D. McAlpine, M. Rosenthal, "Are Patients' Office Visits with Physicians Getting Shorter?" *New England Journal of Medicine* 2001 Jan. 18; Vol. 344, Num. 3:198–204.
6. Bartlett, J., J. Gallant, *2001–2002 Medical Management of HIV Infection*. Baltimore, MD: Johns Hopkins University Division of Infectious Diseases 2001.

Week 2: Learning

1. Smith, R., A. Raymond (Editor). *Encyclopedia of AIDS: A Social, Political, Cultural, and Scientific Record of the HIV Epidemic*. New York: Penguin, 2001.
2. U.S. Department of Health and Human Services. "Guidelines for the Use of Antiretroviral Agents in HIV-Infected Adults and Adolescents." February 04, 2002.

Week 3: Living

1. Canadian Psychiatric Association. *HIV & Psychiatry: A Training and Resource Manual*. Ottawa, Ontario: 2000.
2. Power, R., et al. "Self-disclosure of HIV serostatus in relation to depression and social support." Abstract. XIV International AIDS Conference, Barcelona, Spain, 2002.
3. Medved, W., et al. "Vulnerability of Men Who Have Sex With Men in Disclosing HIV-Positive Status to Sexual Partners and Significant Others: Need for Support and Assistance in Disclosure Decision-Making." XIV International AIDS Conference. Barcelona, Spain; July 7–12, 2002.
4. Logue, K., et al. "Coping with HIV+ Life: Experience of Recent Seroconverters." *The Canadian Journal of Infectious Diseases*, 9 (Suppl. A), March/April 1998.

Week 3: Learning

1. National Institute of Allergy and Infectious Diseases. "The Evidence That HIV Causes AIDS." Updated February 2003. Available at:www.niaid.nih.gov/factsheets/evidhiv.htm.

2. Duesberg, P.D. *Inventing the AIDS Virus*, (Washington: Regnery Publishing, 1996).

Week 4: Living

1. Cauffield, J. "The psychosocial aspects of complementary and alternative medicine." *Pharmacotherapy* 2000 November; 20(11):1289–94.
2. Project Inform. "Herbs, Supplements and HIV." Project Inform Fact Sheet. August 2000. For more information, http://www.projectinform.org.
3. Fairfield, K., et al. "Patterns of use, expenditures, and perceived efficacy of complementary and alternative therapies in HIV-infected patients." *Archives of Internal Medicine* 1998 November 9; 158(20):2257–64.
4. Burack, J., et al. "Pilot randomized controlled trial of Chinese herbal treatment for HIV-associated symptoms." *Journal of Acquired Immune Deficiency Syndromes and Human Retrovirology* 1996 August 1; 12(4):386–93.
5. Risa, K., et al. "Alternative therapy use in HIV-infected patients receiving highly active antiretroviral therapy." *International Journal of STD & AIDS* 2002 Oct; 13(10):706–13.
6. Ernst, E. "The risk-benefit profile of commonly used herbal therapies: Ginkgo, St. John's Wort, Ginseng, Echinacea, Saw Palmetto, and Kava." *Annals of Internal Medicine* 2002 January 1; 136(1):42–53.
7. U.S. Food and Drug Administration. "Kava-Containing Dietary Supplements May Be Associated with Severe Liver Injury." Consumer Advisory. March 25, 2002).
8. Piscitelli. S. "Indinavir Concentrations and St. John's Wort." *The Lancet*, Vol. 355, No. 9203, 12 February 2000.
9. Goldberg, B. *Alternative Medicine: The Definitive Guide*, (Berkeley, California: Celestial Arts, 2002. (yoga: p. 465–473; massage: p. 503; meditation: p. 344–345).
10. Shekelle, P., et al. "Congruence Between Decisions to Initiate Chiropractic Spinal Manipulation for Low Back Pain and Appropriateness Criteria in North America." *Annals of Internal Medicine*, Vol. 129, 1998, pp. 9–17.
11. Shlay, J., et al. "Acupuncture and amitriptyline for pain due to HIV-related peripheral neuropathy: a randomized controlled trial. Terry Beirn Community Programs for Clinical Research on AIDS." *Journal of the American Medical Association* 1998 November 11; 280 (18):1590–5.

Week 4: Learning

1. The New Mexico AIDS InfoNet. "Fact Sheet 125: Viral Load Tests." New Mexico AIDS Education and Training Center, University of New Mexico Health Sciences Center, March 2003.
2. The New Mexico AIDS InfoNet. "Fact Sheet 124: T-Cell Tests." New Mexico AIDS Education and Training Center, University of New Mexico Health Sciences Center, November 2002.
3. U.S. Department of Health and Human Services. "Guidelines for the Use of Antiretroviral Agents in HIV-Infected Adults and Adolescents." February 04, 2002.

Month 2: Living

1. Page-Shafer, K., et al. "Risk of infection attributable to oral sex among men who have sex with men and in the population of men who have sex with men." *AIDS* 2002; 16, 17, 2350–352.
2. Centers for Disease Control & Prevention. "How is HIV passed from one person to another?" Fact Sheet. November, 1998.
3. Page-Shafer, K., et al. "Risk of infection attributable to oral sex among men who have sex with men and in the population of men who have sex with men." *AIDS* 2002; 16, 17, 2350–352.
4. Dillion, B., et al. "Primary HIV Infections Associated with Oral Transmission." Abstract #473, Poster Presentation. Seventh Conference on Retroviruses and Opportunistic Infections, San Francisco, January 30–February 2, 2000.
5. Trust, T. "Oral Sex Issues for Men With HIV." Briefing Sheet. September 2002.
6. Trust, T. "Oral Sex Issues for Women With HIV." Briefing Sheet. September 2002.
7. Trust, T. "Sexually Transmitted Infections: Issue for People with HIV." Briefing Sheet. September 2002.
8. Centers for Disease Control & Prevention. "Can I Get HIV from Having Vaginal Sex?" Fact Sheet. March 2003.
9. Canadian AIDS Society. *Safer Sex Guidelines, Healthy Sexuality and HIV: A Resource Guide for Educators and Counsellors.* Ottawa, 1994.
10. Jost, S., et al. "A Patient with HIV-1 Superinfection." *New England Journal of Medicine* 2002; 347:371.
11. Rhodes, T., L. Cusick. "Accounting for Unprotected Sex: Stories of Agency and Acceptability." *Social Science and Medicine* 2002 July; 55(2):211–26.
12. Mansergh, G., et al. "Barebacking in a Diverse Sample of Men Who Have Sex with Men." *AIDS* 2002 Mar 8; 16:653–9.
13. Castilla, J., et al. "Late Diagnosis of HIV Infection in the Era of Highly Active Antiretroviral Therapy: Consequences for AIDS Incidence." *AIDS* 2002 September 27; 16(14):1945–51.
14. Weller, S., K. Davis, "Condom Effectiveness in Reducing Heterosexual HIV Transmission." Cochrane Database of Systematic Reviews 2002; (1):CD003255.

Month 2: Learning

1. Wald, A., J. Zeh, S. Selke, et al. "Reactivation of genital herpes simplex virus type 2 infection in asymptomatic seropositive persons," *New England Journal of Medicine.* 2000; 342: 844–50.
2. Wald, A., K. Link, "Risk of human immunodeficiency virus infection in herpes simplex virus type-2 seropositive persons: A meta-analysis," *Journal Infectious Disease.* 2002.
3. Schacker, T. "The role of HSV in the transmission and progression of HIV," *Herpes,* 2001.
4. Schacker, T., A. J. Ryncarz, J. Goddard, K. Diem, M. Shaughnessy, L. Corey, "Frequent recovery of HIV-1 from genital herpes simplex virus lesions in HIV-1 infected men," *JAMA* 1998.
5. Conant, M., T. Schacker, R. Murphy, et al. "Valaciclovir versus aciclovir for herpes simplex virus infection in HIV-infected individuals: two randomized trials," *International Journal STD & AIDS* 2002.

6. Centers for Disease Control and Prevention, "Tracking the Hidden Epidemics 2000, Trends in STDs in the United States," 2001.
7. Palefsky, J., "Human papillomavirus-associated malignancies in HIV-positive men and women," *Curr Opin Oncol* 7:437–41, 1995.
8. Minkoff, H., L. Ahdieh, L. Massad, et al. "The effect of highly active antiretroviral therapy on cervical cytologic changes associated with oncogenic HPV among HIV-infected women." *AIDS* 2001.
9. Pfister, H., "Relationship of papillomaviruses to anogenital cancer," *Obstet Gynecol Clin North Am* 14:349–61, 1987.
10. Martins C, "HPV-induced Anal Dysplasia: What Do We Know and What Can We Do About It?" *The Hopkins HIV Report*, May 2001.
11. National Institute of Allergy and Infectious Diseases, "Infection by Closely Related HIV Strains Possible," November 27, 2002, Press release at www.niaid.nih.gov.
12. Lima, M.I.M., V.H. Melo, C. P. Tafuri, et al, for the Research Group Women and HIV, "Risk factors to cervical intraepithelial neoplasia recurrence after loop electrosurgical excision procedure in HIV-1-infected and non-infected women," Abstract of the XVI International AIDS Conference; August 13–18, 2006.
13. Piketty, C., H. Selinger-Leneman, S. Grabar, et al. "Dramatic increase in the incidence of anal cancer despite HAART in the French hospital database of HIV," Abstracts from the XVI International AIDS Conference. August 13–18, 2006.

Month 3: Living

1. National Institutes of Mental Health, "Depression." NIH Publication 2000; No. 00-3561.
2. Eller, L. "Effects of Cognitive-Behavioral Interventions on Quality of Life in Persons with HIV." *International Journal of Nursing Studies* 1999; 36:223–233.
3. May, T., et al. "Characteristics and Causes of Death Among HIV-infected Patients Who had a Good Immunovirologic Response under HAART: French National Survey (Mortalité 2000)." Abstract 913. Tenth Conference on Retroviruses and Opportunistic Infections 2003.
4. Kunches, L., et al. "Mental Health Diagnoses and Medications in HIV Patients Receiving Care in Publicly-funded Clinics." Poster. Ninth International AIDS Conference 2002.
5. Friedwald, V. *Ask the Doctor: Depression*. (Kansas City, Missouri: Andrews McMeel Publishing, 1998).
6. Bonacini, M., M. Puoti. "Hepatitis in Patients with Human Immunodeficiency Virus Infection." *Archives of Internal Medicine* 2000; 160:3365–73.
7. Farber, E., et al. "Resilience Factors Associated with Adaptation to HIV Disease." *Psychosomatics* 2000; 41:140–46.
8. Sherbourne, C., et al. "Impact of Psychiatric Conditions on Health-Related Quality of Life in Persons with HIV Infection." *American Journal of Psychiatry* 2000; 157: 248–54.
9. Ling, S., et al. "Depression, Social Support, and Quality of Life in HIV Patients." Abstract 14343. Twelfth World AIDS Conference 1998.
10. Kelly, B., et al. "Suicidal Ideation, Suicide Attempts, and HIV Infection." *Psychosomatics* 1998; 39: 405–15.

Month 3: Learning

1. National Institutes of Mental Health. "Depression and HIV/AIDS." May 2002. NIH Publication No. 02-5005.
2. Stober, D., et al. "Depression and HIV Disease: Prevalence Correlates and Treatment." *Psychiatric Annals* 27(5): 372–77.
3. Risa, K., et al. "Determinants of Alternative Therapy Use in HIV Infected Patients Receiving HAART." Annual Meeting of the Association of Nurses in AIDS Care. October 2000.
4. Cabaj, R. "Management of Depression and Anxiety in HIV-Infected Patients." *Journal of the International Association of Physicians in AIDS Care.* June 1996.
5. Canadian Psychiatric Association. *HIV & Psychiatry: A Training and Resource Manual.* Ottawa, Ontario: 2000.

Month 4: Living

1. Beckett, M., A. Burnam, R. Collins, D. Kanouse, and R. Beckman, "Substance Use and High-Risk Sex Among People with HIV: A Comparison Across Exposure Groups," *AIDS and Behavior*, Vol. 7, No. 2, June 2003.
2. Turner, B., J. Fleishman, N. Wenger, A. London, M. Burnam, M. Shapiro, E. Bing, M. Stein, D. Longshore, S. Bozzette, "Effects of Drug Abuse and Mental Disorders on Use and Type of Antiretroviral Therapy in HIV-Infected Persons," *Journal General Internal Medicine* 2001. September 16 (9):625–33.
3. Bower M, et al. "HIV-Related Lung Cancer in the Era of Highly Active Antiretroviral Therapy," *AIDS* 17:371, 2003.
4. Diaz, P., M. King, E. Pacht, M. Wewers, J. Gadek, H. Nagaraja, J. Drake, T. Clanton, "Increased Susceptibility to Pulmonary Emphysema Among HIV-Seropositive Smokers," *Ann Internal Medicine* March 7, 2000.
5. Samet, J., and others. "Alcohol consumption and HIV disease progression: Are they related?" *Alcoholism, Clinical and Experimental Research* 27(5): 862–867. May 2003.
6. Abrams, D.I., and others. "Short-term effects of cannabinoids on HIV-1 viral load" Abstract and Late Breaker poster presentation LbPeB 7053 at the XIII International AIDS Conference. July 9–14, 2000.

Month 4: Learning

1. U.S. Department of Health and Human Services, Public Health Service, Substance Abuse and Mental Health Services Administration, Center for Substance Abuse Treatment, "Substance Abuse Treatment for Persons with HIV/AIDS," 2000. Treatment Improvement Protocol Series; no. 37.
2. National Institute on Drug Abuse, National Institutes of Health. "Principles of Drug Addiction Treatment: A Research-Based Guide," NIH Publication No. 00–4180, July 2000.
3. National Institute on Drug Abuse, "An Individual Drug Counseling Approach to Treat Cocaine Addiction," *Therapy Manuals for Drug Addiction.* U.S. Department of Health and Human Services. 2001.
4. Margolin, A., S. Avants, J. Setaro, H. Rinder, L. Grupp, "Cocaine, HIV, and Their Cardiovascular Effects: Is There a Role for ACE-Inhibitor Therapy?" *Drug Alcohol Dependency* December 22, 2000.

5. Beltram, J., M. Park, "HIV Seroprevalence in Cocaine Users Treated at an Atlanta Drug Treatment Center," Georgia Epidemiology Report. Vol. 16, number 6. June 2000.

Month 5: Living

1. Beckett, M., A. Burnam , R. Collins, D. Kanouse, and R. Beckman "Substance Use and High-Risk Sex Among People with HIV: A Comparison Across Exposure Groups," *AIDS and Behavior*, Vol. 7, No. 2, June 2003.
2. U.S. Department of Health and Human Services. Methamphetamine Use, National Survey on Drug Use and Health. NSDUH Report. January 26, 2007.
3. Lee, Steven J. *Overcoming Crystal Meth Addiction: An Essential Guide to Getting Clean*. (Marlowe & Company, 2006).

Month 5: Learning

1. U.S. Department of Health and Human Services. Methamphetamine Use, National Survey on Drug Use and Health. NSDUH Report. January 26, 2007.
2. Roan, S., "Addiction treatment, novel but unproved," *Los Angeles Times*, October 9, 2006.
3. National Institute on Drug Abuse, National Institutes of Health. "Principles of Drug Addiction Treatment: A Research-Based Guide," NIH Publication available at.nida.nih.gov/PODAT/PODATindex.html. 2006.

Month 6: Living

1. Semple, S.J., J. Zians, I. Grant, T.L. Patterson, "Sexual compulsivity in a sample of HIV-positive methamphetamine-using gay and bisexual men," *AIDS Behavior*. September;10(5): 587–98, 2006.
2. Kalichman, S.C., D. Rompa, "The Sexual Compulsivity Scale: Further development and use with HIV-positive persons," *J Pers Assess*. Jun; 76(3):379–95, 2001.
3. Kalichman, S.C., D. Cain, Research Support, U.S. Government, *P.H.S. J Sex Res*. August; 41(3):235–41. 2004.
4. Kalichman, S.C., D. Cain, A. Zweben, G. Swain, "Sensation seeking, alcohol use and sexual risk behaviors among men receiving services at a clinic for sexually transmitted infections," *J Stud Alcohol*. Jul;64(4):564–9. 2003.
5. Lightfoot, M., J. Song, M.J. Rotheram-Borus, P. Newman., "The influence of partner type and risk status on the sexual behavior of young men who have sex with men living with HIV/AIDS," *Journal Acquired Immune Deficiency Syndrome*. Jan 1; 38(1):61–8. 2005.
6. Lambert, S., A. Keegan, J. Petrak., "Sex and relationships for HIV positive women since HAART: A quantitative study," *Sex Transm Infect*. Aug;81(4):284. 2005.
7. Keegan, A., S. Lambert, J. Petrak, "Sex and relationships for HIV-positive women since HAART: A qualitative study," *AIDS Patient Care* October; 19(10):645–54. 2005.

Month 6: Learning

1. Sturm, R., "The Effects of Obesity, Smoking, and Problem Drinking on Chronic Medical Problems and Health Care Costs," *Health Affairs*, 2002; 21(2):245–53.
2. Hodgsona, L., H. Ghattasa, H. Pritchitta, A. Schwenka, L. Payneb, D. Macallana, "Wasting and obesity in HIV outpatients," *AIDS* 2001;15:2341–2.
3. Currier, J., F. Boyd, H. Kawabata, C. Dezii, B. Burtcel, S. Hodder, "Diabetes Mellitus in HIV-Infected Individuals," Poster Presentation, Ninth Conference on Retroviruses and Opportunistic Infections. 2002.
4. Fairfield, K., D. Eisenberg, R. Davis, H. Libman, R. Phillips. "Patterns of use, expenditures, and perceived efficacy of complementary and alternative therapies in HIV-infected patients," *Arch Intern Med.* November 9,1998.
5. Thompson, R.L., C.D. Summerbell CD, L. Hooper, et al. "Dietary advice given by a dietitian versus other health professional or self-help resources to reduce blood cholesterol," *Cochrane Review*, 2001.
6. Romanowski, A., L. Zullig, "Diet Wise, Pound Foolish: Promoted Diets for HIV" AIDS Community Research Initiative of America Update, Spring 2002.
7. Sutinen, J., A. Häkkinen, J. Westerbacka, A. Seppälä-Lindroos, S. Vehkavaara, J. Halavaara, A. Järvinen, M. Ristola, H. Yki-Järvinen, "Increased fat accumulation in the liver in HIV-infected patients with antiretroviral therapy-associated lipodystrophy," AIDS 16(16): 2183–2193; April 2002.
8. Hadigan, C., S. Jeste, E.L. Anderson EJ, et al., "Modifiable dietary habits and their relation to metabolic abnormalities in men and women with human immunodeficiency virus infection and fat redistribution," *Clin Infect Dis.* 2001.
9. Kosmiski, L.A., D.R., Kuritzkes, K.A. Lichtenstein, et al. Fat distribution and metabolic changes are strongly correlated and energy expenditure is increased in the HIV lipodystrophy syndrome. *AIDS*, 2001;15:1993–2000.
10. Dube, M., D. Sprecher, W. Henry, et al. "Preliminary guidelines for the evaluation and management of dyslipidemia in adults infected with human immunodeficiency virus and receiving antiretroviral therapy: Recommendations of the Adult AIDS Clinical Trial Group Cardiovascular Disease Focus Group," *Clin Infect Dis,* 2000.
11. BHIVA Writing Committee. "British HIV Association guidelines for the treatment of HIV-infected adults with antiretroviral therapy." *HIV Med.* 2001.
12. Hooper, L., "Survey of UK dietetic departments: diet in secondary prevention of myocardial infarction." *J Hum Nutr Diet.* 2001.
13. Hooper, L., "Dietary fat intake and prevention of cardiovascular disease: systematic review," *BMJ*, 2001.
14. Egger, M., "HAART and the heart: lipodystrophy and cardiovascular risk," *PRN Notebook.* 2001.
15. Carr, A., K. Samaras, S. Burton, et al. "A syndrome of peripheral lipodystrophy, hyperlipidaemia and insulin resistance in patients receiving HIV protease inhibitors," *AIDS*, 1998. .
16. Wierzbicki, A.S., "Does diet have a role in the treatment of hyperlipidaemia?" *Int J Clin Pract.* 2000.
17. Moyle, G.J., Lloyd M, B. Reynolds, et al. "Dietary advice with or without pravastatin of hypercholesterolaemia associated with protease inhibitor therapy," *AIDS*, 2001.
18. Tang, A., and others. Weight Loss and Survival in HIV-Positive Patients in the Era of Highly Active Antiretroviral Therapy. *Journal of Acquired Immune Deficiency Syndromes*, 2002.

Month 7: Living

1. Shapiro M, Bozzette S, Berry S, Morton S, Leibowitz A, Lefkowitz D, Fleishman J, Arnett R, "The HIV Cost and Services Utilization Study," RAND and the Agency for Health Care Policy and Research. 1999.
2. Shapiro MF, Morton SC, McCaffrey DF, et al. "Variations in the Care of HIV-Infected Adults in the United States." Journal of the American Medical Association 1999.
3. National ADAP Monitoring Project, "Trends in Opportunistic Infection Drug Coverage and Spending," Issue Brief. February 2003.

Month 7: Learning

1. Americans With Disabilities Act of 1990. S. 933.
2. U.S. Equal Employment Opportunity Commission, U.S. Department of Justice
3. Civil Rights Division, "Americans with Disabilities Act: Questions and Answers" www.usdoj.gov/crt/ada/qandaeng.htm.

Month 8: Living

1. U.S. Department of Health and Human Services, Office of AIDS Research Advisory Council, "Guidelines for the Use of Antiretroviral Agents in HIV-1-Infected Adults and Adolescents," May 4, 2006.
2. Hammer, S.M., et al., Treatment for Adult HIV Infection: 2006 Recommendations of the International AIDS Society–USA Panel, *Journal of the American Medical Association*, Vol. 296, No. 7, August 16, 2006.
3. Samet, J., K. Freedberg, M. Stein, R. Lewis, J. Savetsky, L. Sullivan, S. Levenson, R. Hingson, "Trillion Virion Delay: Time From Testing Positive for HIV to Presentation for Primary Care," *Arch Intern Med,* 1998.
4. Yeni, P.G., et al., "Antiretroviral Treatment for Adult HIV Infection in 2002," *JAMA* 2002.
5. Dybul M, et al. "Antiretroviral Therapy for Adults and Adolescents," *MMWR* 2002.

Month 8: Learning

1. U.S. Department of Health and Human Services, Office of AIDS Research Advisory Council, "Guidelines for the Use of Antiretroviral Agents in HIV-1-Infected Adults and Adolescents," May 4, 2006.
2. Hammer, S.M., et al., Treatment for Adult HIV Infection: 2006 Recommendations of the International AIDS Society–USA Panel, *Journal of the American Medical Association*, Vol. 296, No. 7, August 16, 2006.
3. Egger M, et al., "Prognosis of HIV-1-infected Patients Starting Highly Active Antiretroviral Therapy: A Collaborative Analysis of Prospective Studies," *Lancet* 2002.
4. Hadigan, Colleen, and others. "Prediction of Coronary Heart Disease Risk in HIV-Infected Patients with Fat Redistribution," *Clinical Infectious Diseases* 36: 909–16. March 2003.

5. Yeni, P., et al., "Antiretroviral Treatment for Adult HIV Infection in 2002," *JAMA*, 2002.
6. Dybul, M., et al. "Antiretroviral Therapy for Adults and Adolescents," *MMWR*, 2002.
7. U.S. Department of Health and Human Services, "Guidelines for the Use of Antiretroviral Agents in HIV-Infected Adults and Adolescents," February 04, 2002.
8. Robbins, G., et al. "Antiretroviral strategies in naïve HIV+ subjects: comparison of sequential 3-drug regimens," (ACTG 384). *NIAID News,* 2002.
9. Little, S.J., et al., "Antiretroviral Drug Resistance Among Patients Recently Infected with HIV," *N Engl J Med.* 2002.
10. Chambliss, P., et. al. "Once daily HAART: A new paradigm for HIV treatment success," Abstract MoPeB3293. XIV International AIDS Conference. July 7–12, Barcelona, Spain. 2002.

Month 9: Living

1. Tracy Swan, "Care and Treatment for Hepatitis C and HIV Coinfection," U.S. Department of Health and Human Services, Health Resources and Services Administration, HIV/AIDS Bureau, April 2006.
2. Sifakis, F., J. Hylton, D. Celentano, "Hepatitis B and Hepatitis C infections among young men who have sex with men," The Baltimore young men's survey. Abstract. Ninth Conference on Retroviruses and Opportunistic Infections.
3. Mohsen, A., et al. "Progression rate of liver fibrosis in human immunodeficiency virus and hepatitis C virus coinfected patients, UK experience," Abstract MoOrB1057 . XIV International AIDS Conference. Barcelona, Spain, July 7–12, 2002.
4. Consensus Developmental Panel: National Institutes of Health Consensus Developmental Conference Statement: Management of Hepatitis C. Available at www.consensus.nih.gov/cons/116/116cdc_intro.htm.

Month 9: Learning

1. Rodrígueza, M., C. Joan C, "Uncoupling protein 1 gene expression implicates brown adipocytes in highly active antiretroviral therapy-associated lipomatosis," *AIDS*, Vol 18(6) 9 April 2004.
2. Schambelan, M., C. Benson, A. Carr, J. Currier, M. Dube, J. Gerber, S. Grinspoon , C. Grunfeld, D. Kotler., K. Mulligan, W. Powderly, and M. Saag, "Management of Metabolic Complications Associated with Antiretroviral Therapy for HIV-1 Infection: Recommendations on an International AIDS Society-USA Panel," *JAIDS*, Vol. 31, November 1, 2002.
3. Carr, A., K. Samaras, S. Burton, et al. "A syndrome of peripheral lipodystrophy, hyperlipidaemia and insulin resistance in patients receiving HIV protease inhibitors," *AIDS*. 1998.

Month 10: Living

1. Chesney, M. "Adherence to HAART Regimens." *AIDS Patient Care and STDS* 2003 Apr; 17(4): 169–77.

2. Ammassari, A., et al. "Determinants of Non-adherence in a Multicenter Cohort Study of Patients Previously Naïve to Antiretroviral Therapy." Program and Abstracts of the Fifth International Congress on Drug Therapy in HIV Infection, October 2000. Abstract 111.
3. Goujard, C., et al. "Factors Determining Adherence to HAART in a Cohort of 324 HIV-1-Infected Individuals." Program and Abstracts of the Fifth International Congress on Drug Therapy in HIV Infection, October 2000. Abstract 95.

Month 10: Learning

1. Clayton, J., et al, "Gender Differences in HIV Disease Progression," Program and Abstracts of the 13th International AIDS Conference, July 2000, Durban, South Africa, Abstract WePpD1344.

Month 11: Living

1. Cohen-Stuart, J., A. Wensing, and others. "Mechanisms Underlying Transient Relapses ("blips") of Plasma HIV RNA in Patients on HAART." Antiviral Therapy 2000; 5 (Supplement 3):107 and abstract 137 at the 4th International Workshop on HIV Drug Resistance and Treatment Strategies; June 12–16, 2000; Sitges, Spain.
2. Havlir, D. and others. "Prevalence and Predictive Value of Intermittent Viremia in Patients with Viral Suppression." Antiviral Therapy 2000; 5 (Supplement 3):89 and abstract/oral presentation 112 at the 4th International Workshop on HIV Drug Resistance and Treatment Strategies; June 12–16, 2000; Sitges, Spain.

Month 11:Learning

1. Salama, C., M. Policar, C. Cervera, "Knowledge of Genotypic Resistance Mutations Among Providers of Care to Patients with Human Immunodeficiency Virus." Clinical Infectious Diseases 2003; 36:101–4.

Month 12: Living

1. Tuomala, R., et al. "Antiretroviral Therapy During Pregnancy and the Risk of Adverse Outcome." New England Journal of Medicine 2002; 346:1863.
2. Fundaro, C., et al. "Myelomeningocele in a Child with Intrauterine Exposure to Efavirenz." AIDS 2002; 16:299.
3. Minkoff, H. "Ethical Considerations in the Treatment of Infertility in Women with Human Immunodeficiency Virus Infection." The New England Journal of Medicine, 2000 June 8; No. 23, Vol. 342:1748–50.

National Hotlines

HIV AND STDs

HIV/AIDS Information
*Information about HIV/AIDS, TB,
  STDs, referrals, references, workplace issues, and personal questions [CDC]*
(800) 458–5231
http://www.cdc.gov

HIV/AIDS and STD Hotline:
(800) 342–2437
TTY/TDD: (800) 243–7889
Spanish: (800) 344–7432

**Health Information for Sex
Workers:**
Hours 11–6, crisis intervention
(800) 676–4477
http://www.hips.org

National Institutes of Health
Clinical trials information
(800) 243–7644
http://clinicaltrials.gov

LEGAL

**Americans with Disabilities Act
Information and Assistance**
For questions about discrimination
(800) 514–0301
TTY: (800) 514–0383
http://www.ada.gov

Federal Information Center
*For questions about federal agencies,
  programs, benefits, or services*
(800) 688–9889
TTY: (800) 326–2996
http://www.info.gov

Victims of Crime Hotline
*Provides crisis intervention, assis-
  tance with the criminal justice
  process, counseling, and support
  groups*
(800) 394–2255
http://www.ncvc.org

**Center for Medicare and Medicaid
Services**
*Provides information about Medicare,
  Medicaid, billing, benefits, coverage,
  health plan choices, and claims*
(800) 633–4227
TTY: (877) 486–2048
http://www.cms.hhs.gov

GAY AND LESBIAN

Gay and Lesbian Hotline
General questions about gay and lesbian issues
(888) 843–4564
http://www.glnh.org

Pride Institute
Addiction treatment center for gay and lesbian populations
(800) 547–7433
http://www.pride-institute.com

HEMOPHILIA

Hemophilia and AIDS/HIV Network
(800) 424–2634
http://www.hemophilia.org

YOUTH

Child Abuse Hotline
Information about child abuse issues
(800) 422–4453
http://www.childhelp.org

Runaway/Crisis Hotline for Teenagers
24 hour information for adolescents
(800) 621–4000
http://nrscrisisline.org

National Youth Crisis Hotline
Crisis information for youth 17 years and younger
(800) 442–4673

FAMILY

Domestic Violence Hotline
24-hour information, crisis intervention, and referrals to local agencies
(800) 799–7233
http://www.ndvh.org

Rape, Abuse, and Incest National Network Hotline
(800) 656–4673
http://www.rainn.org

Parents Anonymous Help Line
(800) 345–5044
http://www.parentsanonymous.org

NATIVE AMERICANS

National Native American AIDS Prevention Center
(510) 444–2051
http://www.nnaapc.org

WOMEN

Women with HIV Hotline
(800) 554–4876
http://www.women-alive.org

Women's Health Information Center
(800) 994–9662
http://www.4women.gov

Rape, Abuse, and Incest National Network Hotline
(800) 656–4673
http://www.rainn.org

SUICIDE

Suicide Hotline
For crisis calls
(800) 784–2433
http://www.suicidepreventionlifeline.org

HIV/AIDS TREATMENTS

HIV/AIDS Treatment Information Service
Information about HIV medications and clinical trials
(800) 448–0440
http://www.aidsinfo.nih.gov

HIV Treatment Information
Information about HIV medications; calls accepted from incarcerated individuals
(800) 822–7422
http://www.projectinform.org

VETERANS

VA Assistance Service
(800) 827–1000
http://www.va.gov

Mental Health

Mental Health America
*Information on disorders and referrals to
mental health providers*
(800) 969–6642
http://www.nmha.org

**National Mental Health Consumer Self-
Help Clearinghouse**
General inquiries
(800) 553–4539
http://mhselfhelp.org

Substance Abuse/Addictions

**Al-Anon and Alteen Families and Friends
of Alcoholics**
12-step program
(888) 425–2666
http://www.al-anon.org

Sexual Compulsives Anonymous
*12-step program providing information about
local meetings*
(800) 977–4325
http://www.sca-recovery.org

Assisted Recovery
(800) 527–5344
http://www.assistedrecovery.com

Families Anonymous
*12-step program for family members of peo-
ple who may abuse drugs or alcohol*
(800) 736–9805
http://www.familiesanonymous.org

**Clearinghouse for Alcohol and Drug
Information**
(800) 729–6686
http://www.ncadi.samhsa.gov

**National Council on Alcoholism and Drug
Dependence Hopeline**
Information about counseling and treatment
(800) 622–2255
http://ncadd.org

**Drug and Alcohol Treatment Referral
Service**
Provides referrals to local organizations
(800) 662–4357
http://www.samhsa.gov

Cocaine Anonymous Referral Line
*12-step program offering referrals to local
meetings*
(800) 347–8998
http://www.ca.org

**Substance Abuse and Mental Health
Services Administration**
(800) 789–2647
http://www.samhsa.gov

Pride Institute
*Addiction treatment center for gay and les-
bian populations*
(800) 547–7433
http://www.pride-institute.com

Organizations Providing HIV/AIDS Services

Canada

Canadian Aids Society
(800) 499–1986
http://www.cdnaids.ca

United Kingdom

AVERT: Averting HIV and Aids
http://www.avert.org/aidsuk.htm

United States

ALABAMA
Alabama AIDS Hotline
In Alabama: (800) 228–0469
National: (334) 206–5364

AIDS Action Coalition
P.O. Box 2409
Huntsville, AL 35804
(256) 536–4700, (800) 728–3603
http://www.aidsactioncoalition.org

AIDS Alabama
P.O. Box 55703
Birmingham, AL 35255
Local: (205) 324–9822
Statewide Confidential Help Line: (800)
592–2437
http://www.aidsalabama.org

Mobile AIDS Support Services
2054 Dauphin Street
Mobile, AL 36606
(251) 471-5277
http://www.masshelps.org

ALASKA
Alaska AIDS Hotline
In Alaska: (800) 478-2437
National: (907) 276-4880

Alaskan AIDS Assistance Association
1057 W. Fireweed, Suite 102
Anchorage, AK 99503
(907) 263-2050
http://www.alaskanaids.org

Interior AIDS Association
710 Third Avenue
Fairbanks, AK 99707
(907) 452-4222
http://www.interioraids.org

Shanti of Southeast Alaska
P.O. Box 22655
Juneau, AK 99802
(907) 463-5665
http://shanti-seak.org

ARIZONA
Arizona AIDS Hotline
In Arizona: (800) 342-2437
National: (602) 230-5819

AIDS Project Arizona
1427 N. Third Street, Suite 125
Phoenix, AZ 85004
(602) 253-2437
http://www.apaz.org

Casa Gloriosa
3938 E. Grant Road #216
Tucson, AZ 85712
(520) 578-2749
http://parentseyes.arizona.edu/studentpro-
jects/jek/index.html

Children With AIDS Project
P.O. Box 23778
Tempe AZ 85285
(480) 774-9718
http://www.aidskids.org

Southern Arizona AIDS Foundation
375 S Euclid Avenue
Tucson, AZ 85719

(520) 628-7223, (800) 771-9054
http://www.saaf.org

Southwest Behavioral Health Services
Main Office (also locations throughout the
state)
3450 North Third Street
Phoenix, AZ 85012
(602) 265-8338
http://www.sbhservices.org

Tucson Interfaith HIV/AIDS Network
1011 North Craycroft Road #301
Tucson, AZ 85711
(520) 299-6647
http://www.tihan.org

ARKANSAS
Arkansas AIDS Hotline
In Arkansas: (800) 342-2437
National: (501) 661-2408

Arkansas AIDS Foundation
518 East Ninth Street
Little Rock, AR 72202
(501) 376-6299
http://www.araidsfoundation.org

**Arkansas Children's Hospital AIDS
Program**
800 Marshall Street, Slot 401
Little Rock, AR 72202
(501) 364-1100
http://www.archildrens.org

Integrity
6124 North Moor Drive
Little Rock, AR 72204
(501) 614-7200

**Minority AIDS Network/Black Community
Developers**
4000 West 13th Street
Little Rock, AR 72204
(501) 663-9621

Regional AIDS Interfaith Network
614 East Emma Avenue, Suite 209
Springdale, AR 72765
(479) 751-6682

Ryan White Center
510 McLean Street
Little Rock, AR 72203
(501) 376-6299
http://www.angelfire.com/ar2/millscole-
man/rwcbody.html

University of Arkansas for Medical Sciences (UAMS) AIDS Program
4301 W. Markham, Slot 639
Little Rock, AR 72205
(501) 686-7000
http://www.uams.edu

AIDS Outreach of Arkansas
501 Maple Street
North Little Rock, AR 72114
(501) 372-5543, (888) 372-3703
http://www.ashn.org

CALIFORNIA (NORTHERN)

California HIV/AIDS Hotline
TDD: (888) 225-2437
In California: (800) 367-2437
In San Francisco and outside California:
  (415) 863-2437

AIDS Community Research Consortium
1048 El Camino Real, Suite B
Redwood City, CA 94063
(650) 364-6563
http://www.acrc.org

Asian & Pacific Islander Wellness Center
730 Polk Street, Fourth Floor
San Francisco, CA 94109
(415) 292-3400
TTY: (415) 292-3410
http://www.apiwellness.org/contact.html

Genard AIDS Foundation
1630 North Main Street #102
Walnut Creek, CA 94596
(925) 943-2437
http://www.genard.org

AIDS Resources, Information and Services of Santa Clara County
380 North First Street, Suite 200
San Jose, CA 95112
(408) 293-2747
http://www.aris.org

Multicultural AIDS Resource Center
390 Fourth Street
San Francisco, CA 94107
(415) 777-3229

AIDS Emergency Fund
965 Mission Street #630
San Francisco, CA 94103
(415) 558-6999
http://www.aidsemergencyfund.org

AIDS Project of the East Bay
1755 Broadway, Second Floor
Oakland, CA 94612
(510) 663-7979
http://apeb.org

Black Coalition on AIDS
2800 Third Street
San Francisco, CA 94107
(415) 615-9943
TTY: (415) 568-2082
http://www.bcoa.org

Center for AIDS Services
5720 Shattuck Avenue
Oakland, CA 94609
(510) 655-3435
http://vitalcalifornia.org

Native American Health Center
160 Capp Street
San Francisco, CA 94110
(415) 621-8051
http://www.nativehealth.org

Project Inform
205 13th Street, Suite 2001
San Francisco, CA 94103
(415) 558-8669
http://www.projinf.org

Richmond Ermet AIDS Foundation
942 Divisadero Street, Suite 201
San Francisco, CA 94115
(415) 931-0317
http://www.richmondermet.org

San Francisco AIDS Foundation
995 Market Street #200
San Francisco, CA 94103
(415) 487-3000
http://www.sfaf.org

UCSF AIDS Health Project
Client Services
1930 Market Street
San Francisco, CA 94102
(415) 476-3902
http://www.ucsf-ahp.org

UCSF Community Consortium
3180 18th Street, Suite 201
San Francisco, CA 94110
(415) 476-9554
http://www.communityconsortium.org

Center for AIDS Research Education and Services
1500 21st Street
Sacramento, CA 95814
(916) 443-3299
http://www.caresclinic.org

Taylor Family Foundation
5555 Arroyo Road
Livermore, CA 94550
(925) 455-5118
http://www.ttff.org

CALIFORNIA (SOUTHERN)

California HIV/AIDS Hotline
In California: (800) 367-2437
TDD: (888) 225-2437

AIDS Healthcare Foundation
6255 W. Sunset Boulevard, 21st Floor
Los Angeles, California 90028
(323) 860-5200
http://www.aidshealth.org

L.A. Shanti
1616 N. La Brea Ave.
Los Angeles, CA 90028
(323) 962-8197
http://www.lashanti.org

Los Angeles Free Clinic
8405 Beverly Blvd.
Los Angeles, CA 90048
(323) 653-1990
http://www.lafreeclinic.org

Los Angeles Free Clinic
Hollywood Center
6043 Hollywood Blvd.
Los Angeles, CA 90028
(323) 653-1990
http://www.lafreeclinic.org

Los Angeles Free Clinic
Hollywood Wilshire
Health Center
5205 Melrose Avenue
Los Angeles, CA 90038
(323) 653-1990
http://www.lafreeclinic.org

Being Alive
621 N. San Vicente Blvd.
West Hollywood, CA 90069
(310) 289-2551
http://www.beingalivela.org

Camp Pacific Heartland
3310 W. Vanowen Street
Burbank, CA 91505
(818) 260-0372
http://www.hollywoodheart.org

AIDS Project Los Angeles
611 S. Kingsley Drive
Los Angeles, CA 90010
(213) 201-1600
http://www.apla.org

Asian Pacific AIDS Intervention Team
605 W. Olympic Blvd. #605
Los Angeles, CA 90015
(213) 553-1830
http://members.aol.com/apaitmain/apait.htm

Bienestar Latino AIDS Project
4955 Sunset Blvd.
Los Angeles, CA 90027
(323) 660-9680
http://www.bienestar.org

Bienestar Latino AIDS Project
5326 E. Beverly Blvd.
Los Angeles, CA 90022
(323) 727-7896
http://www.bienestar.org

Bienestar Latino AIDS Project
14515 Hamlin Street #100
Van Nuys, CA 91411
(818) 908-3820
http://www.bienestar.org

Bienestar Latino AIDS Project
180 E. Mission Blvd.
Pomona, CA 91766
(909) 397-7660
http://www.bienestar.org

Los Angeles Jewish AIDS Services
P.O. Box 480241
Los Angeles, CA 90048
(323) 655-5330
http://www.projectchickensoup.org

Los Angeles Gay and Lesbian Center
1625 N. Schrader Blvd.
Los Angeles, CA 90028
(323) 993-7400
http://www.lagaycenter.org

Minority AIDS Project
5149 W. Jefferson Blvd.
Los Angeles, CA 90016
(213) 936-4949
http://www.map-usa.org

T.H.E. Clinic for Women
3860 W. Martin Luther King Blvd.
Los Angeles, CA 90008
(323) 295-6571

Watts Health Foundation
3405 West Imperial Highway
Inglewood, CA 90303
(310) 671-3465

Women Alive
1566 Burnside Avenue
Los Angeles, CA 90019
(323) 965-1564
http://www.women-alive.org

Gay & Lesbian Community Center in Long Beach
2017 E. Fourth Street
Long Beach, CA 90814
(562) 434-4455
http://www.centerlb.org

Whittier Rio Hondo AIDS Project
9200 Colima Road #104
Whittier, CA 90605
(562) 698-3850
http://www.wrhap.org

AIDS Assistance Program
1276 N. Palm Canyon, Suite 108
Palm Springs, CA 92262
(760) 325-8481
http://www.aidsassistance.org

Desert AIDS Project
1695 N. Sunrise Way
Palm Springs, CA 92263-2890
(760) 323-2118, (866) 331-3344
http://www.desertaidsproject.org

Being Alive San Diego
Centre Street Office
4070 Centre Street
San Diego, CA 92103
(619) 291-1400
http://www.beingalive.org

Being Alive San Diego
North County Office
804 Pier View Way
Oceanside, CA 92054
(760) 439-6908
http://www.beingalive.org

HIV Consumer Council
Office of Aids Coordination
Health and Human Services Agency
P.O. Box 85524 MS P501-C
San Diego, CA 92186
(619) 293-4700
http://www2.sdcounty.ca.gov/hhsa/Service-
CategoryDetails.asp?ServiceAreaID=27

POZabilities
P.O. Box 34471
San Diego, CA 92163
(619) 282-1866
http://www.sandiegopozabilities.net

Asian Pacific Islander Community AIDS Project
4776 El Cajon Blvd., Suite 204
San Diego, CA 92115
(619) 229-2822
http://www.apicap.org

Sunburst Projects
2 Padre Parkway, Suite 106
Rohnert Park, CA 94928
(707) 588-9477
http://www.sunburstprojects.org

COLORADO

Colorado AIDS Hotline
Denver only: (303) 782-5186
In Colorado: (877) 478-3448

Boulder County AIDS Project
2118 14th Street
Boulder, CO 80302
(303) 444-6121
Spanish: (303) 444-7181
http://www.bcap.org

Northern Colorado AIDS Project
400 Remington Street, Suite 100
Fort Collins, CO 80524
(970) 484-4469
http://www.ncaids.org

Southern Colorado AIDS Project
1301 South Eighth Street, Suite 200
Colorado Springs, CO 80906
(719) 578-9092, (800) 241-5468
http://www.s-cap.org

RESOURCES

CONNECTICUT

AIDS Project Hartford
110 Bartholomew Avenue
Hartford, CT 06106–2241
(860) 951–4833
TTY: (860) 951–4791
http://www.aidsprojecthartford.org

Connecticut AIDS Resource Coalition
20–28 Sargeant Street
Hartford, CT 06105
(860) 761–6699
http://www.ctaidscoalition.org

Mid-Fairfield AIDS Project
16 River Street
Norwalk, CT 06850
(203) 855–9535
http://www.mfap.com

Northwestern Connecticut AIDS Project
100 Migeon Avenue
Torrington, CT 06790
Local: (860) 482–1596
(800) 381–2437
http://www.nwctaids.org

DELAWARE

Delaware AIDS Hotline
In Delaware: (800) 422–0429
National: (302) 652–6776

AIDS Delaware
New Castle County Office
100 West 10th Street, Suite 315
Wilmington, DE 19801
(302) 652–6776
http://www.aidsdelaware.org

AIDS Delaware
Kent & Sussex County Office
706 Rehoboth Avenue, Suite 1
Rehoboth Beach, DE 19971
(302) 226–5350
http://www.aidsdelaware.org

Delaware HIV Consortium
100 West 10th Street, Suite 415
Wilmington, DE 19801
(302) 654–5471
http://www.delawarehiv.org

Sussex County AIDS Committee
P.O. Box 712
Rehoboth Beach, DE 19971
(302) 644–1090
http://www.scacinc.org

DISTRICT OF COLUMBIA

District of Columbia AIDS Information Line
(202) 332–2437
In Metro DC and VA: (800) 322–7432

AIDS Alliance for Children, Youth & Families
1600 K Street N.W., Suite 200
Washington, DC 20006
Local: (202) 785–3564
(888) 917–2437
http://www.aids-alliance.org

Food & Friends
219 Riggs Road N.E.
Washington, DC 20011
(202) 269–2277
http://www.foodandfriends.org

Metro TeenAIDS
651 Penn Avenue S.E.
Washington, DC 20003
(202) 543–9355
http://www.metroteenaids.org

P. L. Active
1772 Church Street N.W.
Washington, DC 20009
(202) 518–8449

National Minority AIDS Council
1931 13th Street N.W.
Washington, DC 20009
(202) 483–6622
http://www.nmac.org

Washington AIDS International Foundation
3224 16th Street N.W.
Washington, DC 20010
(202) 745–0111
http://www.waifaction.org

Whitman-Walker Clinic
1407 S Street N.W.
Washington, DC 20009
(202) 797–3500
TDD: (202) 939–1578
Spanish: (202) 328–0697
Gay/Lesbian Hotline: (202) 833–3234
24-Hour Line: (202) 365–5225
http://www.wwc.org

YouthAIDS
1120 19th Street, Suite 600
Washington, DC 20036
(202) 785–0072
http://projects.psi.org

FLORIDA

Florida AIDS Hotline
In Florida, in English: (800) 352–2437
Haitian Creole: (800) 243–7101
Spanish: (800) 545-SIDA
TTY: (888) 503–7118
National: (850) 681–9131

Care Resource
3510 Biscayne Blvd., Suite 300
Miami, FL 33137
(305) 576–1234
http://www.careresource.org

Joe Logsdon Foundation
2496 Kirkwood Avenue
Naples, FL 34112
(239) 417–8400

League Against AIDS
28 West Flagler Street, Suite 700
Miami, FL 33130
(305) 576–1000
http://www.leagueagainstaids.com

North Central Florida AIDS Network
3615 S.W. 13th Street, Suites 3&4
Gainesville, Florida 32608
(352) 372–4370, (800) 824–6745
http://www.afn.org/~ncfan

Palm Beach County HIV Care Council
4152 West Blue Heron Blvd.
Riviera Beach, Florida 33404
(561) 844–4430
http://www.carecouncil.org

People With AIDS Coalition of Broward
2302 N.E. Seventh Avenue
Ft. Lauderdale, FL 33305
(954) 565–9119

South Beach AIDS Project
1521 Alton Road # 403
Miami Beach, FL 33139
(305) 532–1033
http://www.sobeaids.org

Tampa Bay AIDS Network
North Tampa Office
7402 North 56th Street #101
Tampa, FL 33617
(813) 769–5180
http://www.gcjfs.org/svc-aidsnetwork.htm

GEORGIA

Georgia AIDS Information Line
In Georgia: (800) 551–2728
National: (404) 876–9944

AID Atlanta
1605 Peachtree Street N.W.
Atlanta, GA 30309
(404) 870–7700
TTY/Voice: (404) 870–7773
http://www.aidatlanta.org

AIDS Research Consortium of Atlanta
131 Ponce de Leon Avenue N.E., Suite 130
Atlanta, GA 30308
(404) 876–2317
http://www.aidsresearchatlanta.org

AIDS Survival Project
139 Ralph McGill Blvd., Suite 201
Atlanta, GA 30308
(404) 874 7926
TTY: (404) 524 0464
http://www.aidssurvivalproject.org

Safe Haven
Referrals available by calling:
(229) 225–3997
http://www.safehaveninc.org

HAWAII

Hawaii STD/AIDS Hotlines
In Hawaii: (800) 321–1555
National: (808) 922–1313

Maui AIDS Foundation
1935 Main Street, Suite 101
P.O. Box 858
Wailuku, Maui HI 96793
(808) 242–4900
http://www.mauiaids.org

Maui AIDS Foundation
Moloka'i Office
P.O. Box 341
Kaunakakai, HI 96748
(808) 553–9086
http://www.mauiaids.org

IDAHO

Idaho AIDS Foundation Hotline
In Idaho: (800) 926–2588
National: (208) 321–2777

North Idaho AIDS Coalition
410 Sherman Avenue, Suite 215
Coeur d'Alene, ID 83814
(208) 665-1448
http://nicon.org/niac

South Central Idaho AIDS Coalition
1020 Washington Street N.
Twin Falls, ID 83301
(208) 734-5900

ILLINOIS

In Illinois TTY/TDD: (800) 782-0423
National: (217) 785-7165, (800) 243-2437

AIDS Care
212 E. Ohio
Chicago, Il 60611
(773) 935-4663
http://www.aidscarechicago.org

AIDS Legal Council of Chicago
180 North Michigan Avenue, Suite 2110
Chicago, Illinois 60601
(312) 427-8990
http://www.aidslegal.com

Bethany Place
821 West A Street
Belleville, Illinois 62220
(618) 234-0291
http://www.bethanyplace.org

Better Existence With HIV
1740 Ridge
Evanston, IL 60201
(847) 475-2115
http://www.behiv.org

Central Illinois Friends of PWA
415 St. Marks Court, Suite 504
Peoria, IL 61603
(309) 671-2144
http://www.friendsofpwa.org

Coalition for Positive Sexuality
3712 N. Broadway #191
Chicago, IL 60613
(773) 604-1654
http://www.positive.org

HIV Coalition
990 Criss Circle
Elk Grove Village, IL 60007
(847) 228-5200
http://www.thebody.com/hivco/hivco.html

Howard Brown Health Center
4025 N. Sheridan Road
Chicago, Illinois 60613
(773) 388-1600
http://www.howardbrown.org

Test Positive Aware Network
5537 N. Broadway Street
Chicago, IL 60640
(773) 989-9400
http://www.tpan.com

Jewish AIDS Network—Chicago
3150 Sheridan Road
Chicago, IL 60657
(773) 275-2626
http://www.shalom6000.com/janc.htm

Open Door Clinic
164 Division Street, Suite 607
Elgin, IL 60120
(847) 695-1093
http://www.opendoorclinic.org

Open Door Clinic
Aurora Office
157 S. Lincoln Avenue, Room K
Aurora, IL 60505
(630) 264-1819
http://www.opendoorclinic.org

INDIANA

National AIDS Hotline: (800) 342-2437

Indiana Community AIDS Action Network
3951 North Meridian Street, Suite 200
Indianapolis, IN 46208
(317) 920-3190
http://www.tmg-web.com/hivaids/spns/coopagree_projects/indiana.htm

AIDS Task Force Southeast Central Indiana
1401 Chester Blvd. Jenkins Hall, Fifth Floor
Richmond, IN 47374
(765) 983-3425

Damien Center
26 N. Arsenal Avenue
Indianapolis, IN 46201
(317) 632-0123, (800) 213-1163
http://www.damien.org

Harm Reduction Institute
111 E. 16th Street
Indianapolis, IN 46202
(317) 974-1940

Prevention Point of Indiana
133 West Market Street, Suite 201
Indianapolis, IN 46204
(317) 780-0001

Project AIDS Lafayette
1306 E. Main Street
Crawfordsville, IN 47933
(317) 361-5818

IOWA

Iowa AIDS Hotline
In Iowa: (800) 445-2437
National: (515) 244-6700

Dubuque Regional AIDS Coalition
1454 Iowa Street
Dubuque, IA 52001
(563) 556-6200

Rapids AIDS Project
American Red Cross
6300 Rockwell Drive N.E.
Cedar Rapids, IA 52402
(319) 393-9579
http://www.grantwood-redcross.org/rapidsaids/index.html?aboutra
p.htm&3

KANSAS

Douglas County AIDS Project
United Way Center for Human Resources
2518 Ridge Court, Suite 101
Lawrence, KS 66046
(785) 843-0040
http://www.douglascountyaidsproject.org

Aids Resource Network of Southeast Kansas
P.O. Box 530
201 E. Williams
Pittsburg, KS 66762
(620) 232-8911

KENTUCKY

AIDS Services Center Coalition, Inc.
810 Barret Avenue, Suite 305
Louisville, KY 40204
(502) 574-5490
http://www.asccinc.org

AIDS Interfaith Ministries of Kentuckiana
850 Barret Avenue, Suite 302
Louisville, KY 40204
(502) 574-6085, (502) 574-6086

Family & Children's Counseling Centers
1115 Garvin Place
Louisville, KY 40204
(502) 583-1741

HIV/AIDS Legal Project of the Legal Aid Society
810 Barret Avenue, Suite 301
Louisville, KY 40204
(502) 574-8199

House of Ruth
St. Mathews Campus
607 E. St. Catherine Street
Louisville, KY 40203
(502) 587-5080
http://www.houseofruth.net

Jefferson County Health Department
(502) 574-5600

Jefferson County Health Department Specialty Clinic
850 Barret Avenue, Suite 301
Louisville, KY 40204
(502) 574-6699
http://www.louisvilleky.gov/Health/Specialty-Clinic.htm

Louisville Youth Group
P.O. Box 406764
Louisville, KY 40204
(502) 499-4427
http://www.louisvilleyouthgroup.com

Louisville/Jefferson County Minority AIDS Program
(502) 585-4733
Offices in Louisville, Lexington, Hopkinsville, and Bowling Green

Volunteers of America STOP Program
850 Barret Avenue, Suite 305A
Louisville, KY 40204
(502) 635-1361

WINGS Clinic
(502) 852-2523

AIDS Volunteers
263 N. Limestone Street
Lexington, KY 40507
(859) 225-3000
http://www.aidsvolunteers.org

LOUISIANA

Louisiana AIDS Hotline
In Louisiana: (800) 992–4379
In Louisiana: (504) 821–6050
In Louisiana TDD: (877) 566–9448
National: (785) 296–6036

NO/AIDS Task Force
2601 Tulane Avenue, Suite 500
New Orleans, LA 70119
(504) 821–2601
http://www.noaidstaskforce.org

Food for Friends
2533 Columbus Street
New Orleans, LA 70119
(504) 944–6028

Community Awareness Network
507 Frenchmen Street
New Orleans, LA 70116
(504) 945–4000

Friends for Life
660 North Foster Drive, Building C-100
Baton Rouge, LA 70806
(225) 923–2277

MAINE

Maine AIDS Hotlines:
In Maine: (800) 851–2437
Nationwide: (800) 775–1267

The Maine AIDS Alliance
153 Hospital Street
Pine Tree Store Arboretum
Augusta, ME 04330
(207) 621–2924
http://www.maineaidsalliance.org

MARYLAND

Maryland AIDS Hotline
In Maryland, (Bilingual) (800) 638–6252
In Metro DC. & VA: (800) 322–7432
Hispanic AIDS Hotline: (301) 949–0945
Baltimore only TTY area: (410) 333–2437
National: (410) 767–5013

Deaf AIDS Project
Family Service Foundation
5301 76th Avenue
Landover, MD 20784
(301) 459–2121, (866) 935–4658
TTY: (310) 731–2116
MD Relay: 711
http://www.deafvision.net/dap

Food & Friends (serving Maryland)
219 Riggs Road N.E.
Washington, DC 20011
(202) 269–2277
http://www.foodandfriends.org

Chase Brexton Health Services
Baltimore City
1001 Cathedral Street
Baltimore, MD 21201
(410) 837–2050
http://www.chasebrexton.org

Health Education Resource Organization
Maryland Community Resource Center
1734 Maryland Avenue
Baltimore, MD 21201
(410) 685–1180
http://www.hero-mcrc.org

MASSACHUSETTS

Massachusetts AIDS Hotline
In Massachusetts: (800) 235–2331
National: (617) 536–7733
TTY/TDD: (617) 437–1672
Youth Only AIDS Line toll-free at (800)
    788–1234,
TTY: (617) 450–1427

AIDS Action Committee of Massachusetts
294 Washington Street, Fifth Floor
Boston, MA 02108
(617) 437–6200, (800) 235–2331
TTY: 617–437–1394
http://www.aac.org

AIDS Project Worcester
Worcester Office
85 Green Street
Worcester, MA 01604
(508) 755–3773
http://www.aidsprojectworcester.org

AIDS Project Worcester
South County Office
39 Elm Street
Southbridge, MA 01550
(508) 765–2670
http://www.aidsprojectworcester.org

AIDS Project Worcester
North County Office
14 Manning Avenue, Fourth Floor
Leominster, MA 01453
(978) 466–6868
http://www.aidsprojectworcester.org

Boston Living Center
29 Stanhope Street
Boston, MA 02116
(617) 236-1012
http://www.bostonlivingcenter.org

Common Sensitivity
1 Main Street
Leominster, MA 01453
(978) 840-4673

Community Research Initiative of New England
23 Miner Street
Boston, MA 02215
(617) 778-5454, (888) 253-2712
TTY: 617-778-5460
http://www.crine.org

Community Research Initiative of New England
Springfield Office
780 Chestnut Street, Suite 31
Springfield, MA 01107
(413) 734-2264, (888) 469-6577
http://www.crine.org

North Shore AIDS Health Project
67 Middle Street
Gloucester, MA 01930
(978) 283-0101
http://www.healthproject.org

Positive Directions in Boston
140 Clarendon Street, Suite 805
Boston, MA 02116
(617) 262-3456

Search for a Cure
17 Worcester Street B
Cambridge, MA 02139
(617) 945-5350
http://www.searchforacure.org

TeenAIDS PeerCorps
P.O. Box 7114
Fitchburg, MA 01420
(978) 665-9383
http://www.teenaids.org

MICHIGAN

Michigan AIDS Hotline
In Michigan: (800) 872-2437
TTY/TDD: (800) 332-0849
Spanish: (800) 826-SIDA
Teen Line: (800) 750-TEEN
Health Care Workers: (800) 522-0399
National: (313) 446-9800

AIDS Care Network (Grand Rapids)
207 East Fulton
Grand Rapids, MI 49503
(616) 774-2042
http://www.graceoffice.org

AIDS Partnership Michigan
2751 E. Jefferson, Suite 301
Detroit, MI 48207
(313) 446-9800
http://www.aidspartnership.org

Community AIDS Resource & Education Services
629 Pioneer Street
Kalamazoo, MI 49008
(269) 381-2437, (800) 944-2437
http://www.caresswm.org

Corner Health Center
47 N. Huron Street
Ypsilanti, MI 48197
(734) 484-3600
http://www.cornerhealth.org

Friends Alliance
420 Livernois Street
Ferndale, MI 48220
(313) 279-5302
http://www.friendsalliance.org

HIV/AIDS Resource Center
3075 Clark Road, Suite 203
Ypsilanti, MI 48197
(734) 572-9355, (800) 578-2300

HIV/AIDS Wellness Networks Grand Traverse Area
516 East Eighth Street
Traverse City, MI 49685
(231) 933-0279

Lansing Area AIDS Network
913 West Holmes, Suite 115
Lansing, MI 48910
(517) 394-3719
http://laanonline.org

AIDS Law Project
Wayne County Neighborhood Legal Services
65 Cadillac Square, Suite 3802
Detroit, MI 48226
(313) 962-0466

AIDS Support Group/Tri- Cities
P.O. Box 6361
Saginaw, MI 48603
(517) 758-3877

Alternatives For Girls
903 W. Grand Blvd.
Detroit, MI 48208
(313) 361-4000
http://www.alternativesforgirls.org

American Civil Liberties Union
60 West Hancock
Detroit, MI 48201
(313) 578-6800
http://www.aclumich.org

Bay Area Social Intervention Services
515 Adams Street
Bay City, MI 48708
(989) 894-2991

Black Family Development
2995 E. Grand Blvd.
Detroit, MI 48202
(313) 758-0150
http://www.blackfamilydevelopment.org

Children's Immune Disorder
16888 Greenfield
Detroit, MI 48235-3707
(313) 837-7800

Community Health Awareness Group
1300 W. Fort Street
Detroit, MI 48226
(313) 963-3434

Community Recover Services
711 N. Saginaw, Suite 323
Flint, MI 48503
(810) 238-2068

Detroit American Indian Health and Family Services
4880 Lawndale
Detroit, MI 48210
(313) 846-3781

Detroit Central City Community Mental Health
10 Peterboro
Detroit, MI 48201
(313) 831-3160
http://www.dcccmh.org

Hemophilia Foundation of Michigan
1921 W. Michigan Avenue
Ypsilanti, MI 48197
(734) 544-0015
http://www.hfmich.org

Hispanics Against AIDS
730 Grandville
Grand Rapids, MI 49503
(616) 742-0200

HIV/AIDS Network and Direct Services
708 Jackson Street, Suite 2
Post Office Box 533
Petoskey, MI 49770
(231) 348-6460, (888) 526-9213

HIV/AIDS Services
343 Atlas Avenue
Grand Rapids, MI 49506
(616) 456-9063
http://www.hasinc.org

Latino Family Services
3815 West Fort Street
Detroit, MI 48216
(313) 841-7380

Muskegon Area AIDS Resource Services
1095 Third Street, Suite 221
Muskegon, MI 49441
(231) 722-2437

Neighborhood Services Department
Drug Treatment Program
5031 Grandy Avenue
Detroit, MI 48211
(313) 267-6718

Tribal Health and Human Services
2864 Ashmun Street
Sault Ste. Marie, MI 49783
(906) 632-5274

University of Michigan HIV/AIDS Treatment Program
Department of Internal Medicine
3120 Taubman Center
Ann Arbor, MI 48109
(734) 763-9227
http://www.med.umich.edu/intmed/infec-
tious/hiv/index.htm

MINNESOTA

Minnesota AIDS Line
In Minnesota: (800) 248-2437
National: (612) 373-2437

The Aliveness Project
730 East 38th Street
Minneapolis, MN 55407
(612) 822-7946
http://www.aliveness.org

Delaware Street Clinic
University of Minnesota Medical Center
516 Delaware Street S.E.
Clinic 6B, Sixth Floor
Philips-Wangensteen
Minneapolis, MN 55455
(612) 625-4680

Minnesota AIDS Project
1400 Park Avenue S.
Minneapolis, MN 55404
(612) 341-2060
http://www.mnaidsproject.org

Rural AIDS Action Network
208 Second Street N.E.
Little Falls, MN 56345
(320) 631-0404, (800) 966-9735
http://www.raan.org

Youth and AIDS Projects
University of Minnesota
428 Oak Grove Street
Minneapolis, MN 55403
(612) 627-6820
http://www.yapmn.com

MISSISSIPPI

Mississippi AIDS Hotline
In Mississippi: (800) 826-2961
National: (601) 576-7723

Coastal Family Health Services
1046 Division Street
Biloxi, MS 39530
(228) 374-2494
http://www.coastalfamilyhealth.com

South Mississippi AIDS Task Force
2756 Fernwood Road
Biloxi, MS 39531
(228) 385-1214, (800) 826-2961
http://www.smatf.com

DePorres Health Center
411 Poplar Street
Marks, MS 38646
(662) 326-9232

G. A. Carmichael Family Health Center
P.O. Box 588
1668 West Peace Street
Canton, MS 39046
(601) 859-5213
http://gacfhc.org

Aaron E. Henry Community Health Center
P.O. Box 1216
Clarksdale, MS 38614
(662) 624-4292

Jefferson Comprehensive Health Center
P.O. Box 98
Fayette, MS 39069
(601) 786-3475

Magnolia Medical Clinic
1413 Strong Avenue
Greenwood, MS 38930
(662) 459-1207

Southeast Mississippi Rural Health Initiative
P. O. Box 1729
Hattiesburg, MS 39403
(601) 545-8700

Building Bridges, Inc.
2147 Henry Hill Drive, Suite 206
Jackson, MS 39204
(601) 922-0100
http://www.bbims.org

Catholic Charities
200 North Congress, Suite 101
Jackson, MS 39201
(601) 355-8634
http://www.catholiccharitiesjackson.org

Central Mississippi Circle of Care
350 W. Woodrow Wilson, Suite 751
Jackson, MS 39213
(601) 815-1323

Episcopal AIDS Committee
P. O. Box 55803
Jackson, MS 39216
(601) 936-6780
http://www.neac.org

Jackson State University
National Alumni AIDS Prevention
P. O. Box 18890
1400 J. R. Lynch
Jackson, MS 39217
(601) 968-2512

Mississippi State Department of Health
HIV/AIDS Prevention
570 E. Woodrow Wilson, Suite 350
P. O. Box 1700
Jackson, MS 39215
(601) 576-7723

Project Connect AIDS Service Organization
350 W. Woodrow Wilson, Suite 3210
Jackson, MS 39213
(601) 981-1700

University of Mississippi Medical Center
Infectious Diseases Department
2500 North State Street
Jackson, MS 39216
(601) 984-5552

University of Mississippi Pediatric AIDS
2500 North State Street
Jackson, MS 39216
(601) 984-5206

VA Medical Center
PWA Support Group
1500 E. Woodrow Wilson Drive
Jackson, MS 39216
(601) 362-4471

Greater Meridian Health Clinic
2701 Davis Street
Meridian, MS 39301
(601) 693-0118
http://www.gmhcinc.org

Sharp Family Care Center
P.O. Drawer 32
Tylertown, MS 39667
(601) 876-4926

Sacred Heart Southern Mission
6144 Hwy 61 North, Box 5
Walls, MS 38680
(800) 232-9079
http://shl.convio.net

MISSOURI

Missouri AIDS Information Line
National: (800) 533-2437

AIDS Foundation of St. Louis
2340 Hampton Avenue, Suite 1
St. Louis, MO 63139
(314) 367-7273
http://www.aidstl.org

MONTANA

Montana AIDS PROGRAM
In Montana: (800) 233-6668
National: (406) 444-3565
Eastern Montana AIDS Hotline: (800) 675-2437

Western Montana AIDS Hotline: (800) 663-9002

Butte AIDS Support Services
P.O. Box 382
Butte, MT 59703
(406) 496-6125
http://www.buttebass.org

Falls AIDS Network
2611 10th Avenue South,
P.O. Box 220
Great Falls, MT 59405
(406) 791-9080

Flathead AIDS Council
723 Fifth Avenue East
Kalispell, MT 59901
(406) 752-5500
http://www.montanaweb.com/fhaids

Lewis and Clark AIDS Project
P.O. Box 832
Helena, MT 59624
(406) 447-1322

Mission Valley AIDS Council
802 Main Street
Polson, MT 59860
(406) 883-7314

Missoula AIDS Council
127 N. Higgins, Suite 207
Missoula, MT 59802
(406) 543-4770

Montana Migrant Health Project
3318 Third Avenue N., Suite 100
Billings, MT 59101-1900
(406) 248-3149
http://www.mtpca.org/mtmigrant.htm

PRIDE!
P.O. Box 775
Helena, MT 59624
(800) 610-9322, (406) 442-9322
http://www.gaymontana.com/pride

Ravalli County HIV/AIDS Education and Prevention Council
P.O. Box 190
Stevensville, MT 59870
(406) 777-3646

AIDS Network of Southern Montana
321 E. Main Street, Suite 326
Bozeman, MT 59715
(406) 582-1110

Valley County AIDS Task Force
501 Court House Square, Box 11
Glasgow, MT 59230
(406) 228-8221

Wheatland County AIDS Task Force
Wheatland Memorial Hospital
53 Third Street N.W.
Harlowton, MT 59036
(406) 632-4351

Yellowstone AIDS Project
2906 First Avenue N., Suite 200
Billings, MT 59103
(406) 245-2029
http://www.yapmt.org

NEBRASKA
Nebraska AIDS Hotline
National: (800) 782-2437

Nebraska AIDS Project
Omaha & Watanabe Wellness Center
139 S. 40th Street
Omaha, NE 68131
(402) 552-9260
http://www.nap.org

Nebraska AIDS Project
Lincoln Office
2147 S. 15th Street
Lincoln, NE 68502
(402) 476-7000
http://www.nap.org

Nebraska AIDS Project
Norfolk Office
107 S. Eighth Street
Norfolk, NE 68701
(402) 370-3900
http://www.nap.org

Nebraska AIDS Project
Kearney Office
P.O. Box 2378
11 W Railroad Street
Kearny, NE 68848
(308) 338-0527
http://www.nap.org

Nebraska AIDS Project
Scottsbluff Office
4500 Ave I
P.O. Box 1500
Scottsbluff, NE 69361
(308) 635-3807
http://www.nap.org

NEVADA
Nevada AIDS Information Line
In Nevada: (800) 842-2437
National: (775) 684-5900

Aid for AIDS of Nevada
2300 S. Rancho Drive, Suite 211
Las Vegas, NV 89102
(702) 382-2326
http://www.afanlv.org

Golden Rainbow
3233 W. Charleston Blvd., Suite 108
Las Vegas, NV 89102
(702) 384-2899
http://www.goldenrainbow.org

Northern Nevada H.O.P.E.S
P.O. Box 6420
Reno, NV 89513
(775) 348-2893
http://www.nnhopes.org

NEW HAMPSHIRE
New Hampshire AIDS Hotline
In New Hampshire: (800) 752-2437
National: (603) 271-4502

**Chronic Conditions Information Network
of Vermont and New Hampshire:
HIV/AIDS**
P.O. Box 3
Cavendish, VT 05142
(802) 226-7807
http://www.cc-info.net/hiv/hiv_aids.html

NEW JERSEY
New Jersey AIDS Hotline
In New Jersey: (800) 624-2377 (24 hrs, 7
days)
TTY/TDD: (201) 926-8008
National: (973) 926-7443

AIDS Coalition of Southern New Jersey
100 Essex Avenue, Suite 300
Bellmawr, NJ 08031
(856) 933-9500
http://www.acsnj.org

Hyacinth AIDS Foundation
317 George Street, Suite 203
New Brunswick, NJ 08901
(732) 246-0204
Hotline in NJ/TDD: 1-800-433-0254
Outside of NJ: (732) 246-0204

RESOURCES

National Pediatric & Family HIV Resource Center
University of Medicine & Dentistry of New Jersey
30 Bergen Street—ADMC #4
Newark, NJ 07103
(973) 972–0410, (800) 362–0071
http://www.umdnj.edu

Buddies of New Jersey
Franklin A. Smith Resource Center
149 Hudson Street
Hackensack NJ 07601
(201) 489–2900, (800) 508–7577
http://www.njbuddies.org

South Jersey AIDS Alliance
19 Gordon's Alley
Atlantic City, NJ 08401
(609) 347–1085
http://www.southjerseyaidsalliance.org

Good Shepherd Community Services
1576 Palisade Avenue
Ft. Lee, NJ 07024
(201) 461–7260
http://home.earthlink.net/~-mauel/GoodShepherd.html

Mercer County HIV Consortium
447 Bellevue Avenue
Trenton, NJ 08618
(609) 278–9555

Middlesex County HIV Resource Center
275 Hobart Street
Perth Amboy, NJ 08861
(732) 442–6225

Monmouth-Ocean HIV Care Consortium
625 Bangs Avenue
Asbury Park, NJ 07712
(732) 505–5122

Passaic County AIDS Resource Center
100 Hamilton Plaza, Room 707
Paterson, NJ 07505
(973) 742–6742

Somerset-Hunterdon HIV Care Consortium
95 Veteran's Memorial Drive
Somerville, NJ 08876
(908) 704–9641

South Jersey Council on AIDS
120 White Horse Pike, Suite 110
Haddon Heights, NJ 08035
(856) 547–6600

HIV Care Consortium/Resource Center
16 South Ohio Avenue
Atlantic City, NJ 08401
(609) 441–8181

Union County HIV Consortium
80 West Grand Street, Lower Level
Elizabeth, NJ 07202
(908) 352–7700

NEW MEXICO

New Mexico AIDS Hotline
In New Mexico: (800) 545–2437
National: (505) 476–3612

Camino de Vida
2805 Doral Court
P.O. Drawer 2827
Las Cruces, NM 88004
(505) 532–0202, (800) 687–0850
http://www.caminodevida.org

AIDS Law Panel
P.O. Box 22251
Santa Fe, NM 84502
(505) 982–2021, (800) 982–2021

Southwest Comprehensive AIDS-Care Center
649 Harkle Road, Suite E
Santa Fe, NM 87505
(505) 989–8200, (888) 320–8200
http://www.southwestcare.org

HIV/AIDS Support
(505) 521–4387

NEW YORK

HIV counseling hotline: (800) 872–2777
National: (716) 845–3170
Information hotline: (800) 541–2437
Spanish hotline: (800) 233-SIDA

AIDS Treatment Data Network
611 Broadway, Suite 613
New York, NY 10012
(212) 260–8868
NY only: (800) 734–7104
http://www.atdn.org

Gay Men's Health Crisis
119 West 24th Street
New York, NY 10011
(212) 367–1000
http://www.gmhc.org

Long Island Association for AIDS Care, Inc.
P.O. Box 2859
Huntington Station, New York 11746
(631) 385-2451
http://www.liaac.org

Task Force on AIDS of New York State
Psychological Association
(212) 459-4167

Hispanic AIDS Forum
Manhattan Office
213 W. 35th Street, 12th Floor
New York, NY 10001
(212) 868-6230
http://www.hafnyc.org

Hispanic AIDS Forum
Queens Office
62-07 Woodside Avenue, Third Floor
Woodside, NY 11377
(718) 803-2766
http://www.hafnyc.org

Hispanic AIDS Forum
Bronx Office
886 Westchester Avenue
Bronx, NY 10459
(718) 328-4188
http://www.hafnyc.org

AIDS Council of Northeastern New York
927 Broadway
Albany, NY 12207
(518) 434-4686, (800) 660-6886
http://www.aidscouncil.org

AIDS Council of Northeastern New York
Glens Falls
21 Bay Street, Suite 305
Glens Falls, NY 12801
(518) 743-0703
http://www.aidscouncil.org

AIDS Council of Northeastern New York
Hudson Office
Fairview Plaza
160 Fairview Avenue
Hudson, NY 12534
(518) 828-3624
http://www.aidscouncil.org

AIDS Council of Northeastern New York
Troy Office
392 Second Street
Troy, NY 12180
(518) 272-2308
http://www.aidscouncil.org

AIDS Council of Northeastern New York
Schenectady Office
434 Franklin Street
Schenectady, NY 12305
(518) 346-9272
http://www.aidscouncil.org

AIDS Council of Northeastern New York
Plattsburgh Office
202 Cornelia Street
P.O. Box 903
Plattsburgh, NY 12901
(518) 563-2437
http://www.aidscouncil.org

AIDS Community Services of Western New York
206 South Elmwood Avenue
Buffalo, New York 14201
(716) 847-2441
http://www.aidscommunityservices.com

AIDS-Related Community Services
40 Saw Mill River Road
Hawthorne, NY 10523
(914) 345-8888
http://arcs.org

AIDS Center of Queens County
97-45 Queens Blvd., 12th Floor
Rego Park, NY 11374
(718) 896-2500
http://www.acqc.org

Bronx AIDS Services
540 E. Fordham Road
Bronx, NY 10408
(718) 295-5605
http://www.basnyc.org

Brooklyn AIDS Task Force
502 Bergen Street
Brooklyn, NY 11217
(718) 622-2910
http://www.batf.net

AIDS Rochester
Main Office
1350 University Avenue
Rochester, NY 14607
(585) 442-2220
http://www.aidsrochester.org

AIDS Rochester
Finger Lakes Office
605 W. Washington Street
Geneva, NY 14456
(315) 781-6303
http://www.aidsrochester.org

AIDS Rochester
Southern Tier Office
122 Liberty Street
P.O. Box 624
Bath, NY 14810
(607) 776–9166
http://www.aidsrochester.org

AIDS Community Resources of Central New York
Main Office (Syracuse)
627 W. Genesee Street
Syracuse, NY 13204
(315) 475–2430

AIDS Community Resources of Central New York
Utica Office
1119 Elm Street
Utica, NY 13501
(315) 793–0661

AIDS Community Resources of Central New York
Oswego Office
10 George Street
Oswego, NY 13126
(315) 343–7778

AIDS Community Resources of Central New York
Watertown Office
165 Mechanic Street
Watertown, NY 13601
(315) 785–8222

AIDS Community Resources of Central New York
Canton Office
7 Main Street
Canton, NY 13617
(315) 386–4493

AIDS Community Resources of Central New York
Auburn Office
27 E. Genesee Street
Auburn, NY 13021
(315) 253–7184

Southern Tier AIDS Program
Johnson City Location
122 Baldwin Street
Johnson City, NY 13790
(607) 798–1706
http://www.stapinc.org

Southern Tier AIDS Program
Oneonta Location
31 Main Street
Oneonta, NY 13820
(888) 895–7264
http://www.stapinc.org

Southern Tier AIDS Program
Elmira Location
911 Stowell Street
Elmira, NY 14901
(888) 564–5693
http://www.stapinc.org

Staten Island AIDS Task Force
25 Hyatt Street
Staten Island, NY 10301
(718) 448–8802

Mother's Voices
165 W. 46th Street, Suite 701
New York, NY 10036
(212) 730–2777

Children's Hospital at Montefiore Medical Center Adolescent AIDS Program
111 E. 210th Street
Bronx, NY 10467
(718) 882–0232, (718) 882–0432
http://www.adolescentaids.org

Momentum AIDS Project
322 Eighth Avenue
New York, NY 10001
(212) 691–8100
http://www.momentumaidsproject.org

Coalition for the Homeless
129 Fulton Street
New York, NY 10038
(212) 776–2000
http://www.coalitionforthehomeless.org

Harlem United Community AIDS Center
123–125 W. 124th Street
New York, NY 10027
(212) 531–1300
http://www.harlemunited.org

The Osborne Association AIDS in Prison Project
809 Westchester Avenue
Bronx, NY 10455
(718) 842–0500
http://www.osborneny.org

New York State Office of AIDS Discrimination Issues
(800) 523–2437

Legal Action Center
225 Varick Street
New York, NY 10014
(212) 243-1313
http://www.lac.org

New York City Gay and Lesbian Anti-Violence Project
240 West 35th Street, Suite 200
New York, NY 10001
(212) 714-1184
TTY: (212) 714-1134
Bilingual Hotline: (212) 714-1141
http://www.avp.org

National AIDS Treatment Advocacy Project
580 Broadway, Suite 1010
New York, NY 10012
(212) 219-0106, (888)-266-2827
http://www.natap.org

HIV Law Project
841 Broadway, Suite 608
New York, NY 10003
(212) 674-7590

Tzvi Aryeh AIDS Foundation
P.O. Box 150
Cathedral Station
New York, NY 10025
(212) 866-6306

Friends in Deed
594 Broadway, Suite 706
New York, NY 10012
(212) 925-2009
http://www.friendsindeed.org

Identity House
39 West 14th Street, Suite 205
New York, NY 10011
(212) 243-8181
http://www.identityhouse.org

ADAP Plus (Primary Care)
(800) 542-2437

AIDS Drug Assistance Program
Empire Station
P.O. Box 2052
Albany, NY 12220
(800) 542-2437

Experimental Treatments Infoline
(800) 633-7444

NORTH CAROLINA

North Carolina AIDS Hotline
In North Carolina: (800) 342-2437
National: (919) 733-3039

AIDS Community Residence Association
P.O. Box 25265
Durham, NC 27702-5265
(919) 956-7901
http://www.acra-org.com

Baptist AIDS Partnership of North Carolina
P.O. Box 1318
Wake Forest, NC 27588-1318
(919) 554-3220

Piedmont HIV Health Care Consortium
Piedmont Consortium
331 W. Main Street, Suite 405
Durham, NC 27701
(919) 682-3998, (800) 272-9610
http://www.phicas.org

Metrolina AIDS Project
P.O. Box 32662
Charlotte, NC 28232
(704) 333-1435
http://www.metrolinaaidsproject.org

NORTH DAKOTA

North Carolina AIDS Hotline
In North Carolina: (800) 472-2180
National: (701) 328-2378

North Dakota HIV/AIDS Program
600 E. Boulevard Avenue, Dept. 301
Bismark, ND 58505
(701) 328-2378
http://www.ndhiv.com

OHIO

Ohio AIDS Hotline
In Ohio: (800) 332-2437
In Ohio TTY/TDD: (800) 332-3889
National: (614) 466-6374

AIDS Resource Center Ohio
The Kuhns Building 1183
15 W. Fourth Street, Suite 200
Dayton, OH 45402
(937) 461-2437
http://www.afmv.org

RESOURCES

AIDS Taskforce of Greater Cleveland
3210 Euclid Avenue
Cleveland, OH 44115
(216) 621-0766
http://www.aidstaskforce.org

AIDS Volunteers of Cincinnati
220 Findlay Street
Cincinnati, OH 45210
(513) 421-2437
http://www.avoc.org

Caracole
1821 Summit Road, Suite 001
Cincinnati, OH 45237
(513) 761-1480
http://www.caracole.org

The Columbus AIDS Task Force
1751 E. Long Street
Columbus, OH 43203
(614) 299-2437
http://www.catf.net

Ohio AIDS Coalition
48 W. Whittier Street
Columbus, OH 43206
(614) 444-1683, (800) 226-5554
http://www.ohioaidscoalition.org

Project Open Hand-Columbus
1699 W. Mound Street
Columbus, OH 43223
(614) 298-8334
http://www.projectopenhand-columbus.org

Union County AIDS Task Force
P.O. Box 517
Marysville, OH 43040
(937) 642-0801, (888) 333-9461

OKLAHOMA
Oklahoma AIDS Hotline
In Oklahoma: (800) 535-2437
National: (918) 834-4194

Ahalaya Project/NNAAPC
1211 N. Shartel, Suite 404
Oklahoma City, OK 73103
(405) 235-9988
http://www.nnaapc.org

CarePoint, Consortium of AIDS Resources & Education
1200 N. Walker, Suite 500
Oklahoma City, OK 73103
(405) 232-2437
Outside OKC: (800) 285-2273

Oklahoma City Clinic
701 N.E. 10th Street
Oklahoma City, OK 73104
(405) 280-5700
http://www.okcclinic.com

Red Rock Behavioral Health Services
4400 North Lincoln Blvd.
Oklahoma City, OK 73105
(405) 424-7711
http://www.red-rock.com

Oklahoma Infants Assistance Program
CHO 3B 3406
940 N.E. 13th Street
Oklahoma City, OK 73117
(405) 271-8858
http://ccan.ouhsc.edu/infantparenting.asp

Tulsa C.A.R.E.S.
3507 E. Admiral Place
Tulsa, OK 74115
(918) 834-4194, (800) 474-4872
http://www.tulsacares.org

OREGON
Oregon AIDS Hotline
Area codes 503, 206 and 208: (800) 777-2437
Voice & TTY: (503) 223-2437
National: (503) 223-2437

AIDS Educational Council of Eastern Oregon
P.O. Box 2901
La Grande, OR 97850
(541) 962-7048, (888) 883-5423
http://www.eoni.com/~eastlg/index.html

Cascade AIDS Project (Portland)
620 S.W. Fifth Avenue, Suite 300
Portland, OR 97204
(503) 223-5907
http://www.cascadeaids.org

Oregon Public Health Services
800 N.E. Oregon, Suite 930
Portland, OR 97232
(503) 731-4000
http://www.oregon.gov

Portland Area HIV Services Planning Council
3653 S.E. 34th Avenue
Portland, OR 97202
(503) 988-3030
http://hivportland.org

PENNSYLVANIA

Pennsylvania AIDS Hotline
In Pennsylvania: (800) 662–6080
National: (717) 783–0573

ActionAIDS (Central Office)
1216 Arch Street, Sixth Floor
Philadelphia, PA 19107
(215) 981–0088
http://www.actionaids.org

ActionAIDS (North Office)
2641 N. Sixth Street
Philadelphia, PA 19133
(215) 291–9700
http://www.actionaids.org

ActionAIDS (West Office)
3901 Market Street
Philadelphia, PA 19107
(215) 387–6055
http://www.actionaids.org

Washington West Project
1201 Locust Street
Philadelphia, PA 19107
(215) 985–9206

Berks AIDS Network
429 Walnut Street
P.O. Box 8626
Reading, PA 19603
(610) 375–6523
http://www.berksaidsnetwork.org

Chester County AIDS Support Services
31 S. 10th Avenue, Suite 2
Coatesville, PA 19320
(610) 466–7848

AIDS Library
1233 Locust Street, Second Floor
Philadelphia, PA 19107
(215) 985–4851
http://www.aidslibrary.org

Pittsburgh AIDS Task Force
905 West Street, Fourth Floor
Pittsburgh, PA 15221
(412) 242–2500
http://www.patf.org

Shepherd Wellness Community
4800 Sciota Street
Pittsburgh, PA 15224
(412) 683–4477
http://www.swconline.org

Siloam Ministries
1133 Spring Garden Street
Philadelphia, PA 19123–3315
(215) 765–6633
http://www.siloamministries.org

Southwestern Pennsylvania AIDS Planning Coalition
201 S. Highland Avenue, Suite 101
Pittsburgh, PA 15206
(412) 363–1022, (412) 363–5776, (877) 732–0401
http://www.swpapc.org

AIDS Law Project of Pennsylvania
1211 Chestnut Street, Suite 600
Philadelphia, PA 19107
(215) 587–9377
http://www.aidslawpa.org

AIDS Services in Asian Communities
1201 Chestnut Street, Suite 501
Philadelphia, PA 19107
(215) 563–2424
http://www.critpath.org/asiac

AIDS Treatment Information Service
1233 Locust Street, Fifth Floor
Philadelphia, PA 19107
(800) 873–2812
http://www.aidsnews.org

AIDS Working Groups of Religious Society of Friends
1515 Cherry Street
Philadelphia, PA 19102
(215) 241–7000
http://www.pym.org/peace-and-concerns/aids.html

Albert Einstein Immunodeficiency Center
1335 Tabor Road, Suite 310
Philadelphia, PA 19141
(215) 224–5623

BEBASHI (Blacks Educating Blacks About Sexual Health Issues)
1217 Spring Garden Street, First Floor
Philadelphia, PA 19123
(215) 769–3561
http://www.bebashi.org

Best Nest
1709 Washington Avenue
Philadelphia, PA 19146
(215) 546–8060
http://www.bestnest.org

We Care HIV AIDS Support Network
P.O. Box 1013
Wilkes-Barre, PA 18703
(570) 824–1007
http://www.wecarewb.org

RHODE ISLAND
Rhode Island AIDS Hotline
National: (800) 726–3010

AIDS Care Ocean State
18 Parkis Avenue
Providence, RI 02907
(401) 521–3603
http://www.aidscareos.org

SOUTH CAROLINA

South Carolina AIDS Hotline
In South Carolina: (800) 322–2437
National: (803) 898–0749

AIDS Council of Gaston County
991 West Hudson Blvd.
Gastonia, NC 28053
(704) 853–5101

Catawba Care Coalition
1151 Camden Avenue
Rock Hill, SC 29732
(803) 909–6363
http://www.catawbacare.org

SOUTH DAKOTA

South Dakota AIDS Hotline
In South Dakota: (800) 592–1861
National: (605) 773–3737

TENNESSEE
Tennessee AIDS Hotline
In Tennessee: (800) 525-AIDS
National: (615) 741–7500

Chattanooga CARES
P.O. Box 4497
Chattanooga, TN 37405
(423) 265–2273
http://www.chattanoogacares.org

Hope Center
1901 Clinch Avenue
Knoxville, TN 37916
(865) 541–3767
http://hopecenterknox.org

Nancy's House
P.O. Box 5086
Cleveland, TN 37320
(423) 559–8592
http://www.nancyshouse.org

Nashville CARES
501 Brick Church Park Drive
Nashville, TN 37207
(800) 845–4266
http://www.nashvillecares.org

TEXAS
Texas AIDSLINE
In Texas: (800) 299–2437
National: (572) 490–2505

AIDS Foundation Houston
3202 Weslayan Annex
Houston, TX 77027
(713) 623–6796
http://www.aidshelp.org

**AIDS Outreach Center of Tarrant County
(Fort Worth)**
801 West Cannon
Fort Worth, TX 76104
(817) 335–1994
http://www.aoc.org

**AIDS Outreach Center of Tarrant County
(Arlington)**
401 W. Sanford, Suite 1100
Arlington, TX 76011
(817) 275–3311
http://www.aoc.org

**AIDS Outreach Center of Tarrant County
(Southeast)**
2516 Oakland Blvd., Suite 11
Fort Worth, TX 76103
(817) 535–1113
http://www.aoc.org

AIDS Resource Center of Dallas
2701 Reagan Street
P.O. Box 190869
Dallas, TX 75219
(214) 528–0144
http://www.resourcecenterdallas.org/arc.html

AIDS Services of Austin
P.O. Box 4874
Austin, TX 78765
(512) 458–2437
http://www.asaustin.org

AIDS Services of North Texas (Denton–Main Office)
4210 Mesa Drive
Denton, TX 76207
(940) 381–1501, (800) 974–2437
http://www.aidsntx.org

AIDS Services of North Texas (Plano)
1316 14th Street
Plano, TX 75074
(972) 424–1480, (800) 339–2437
http://www.aidsntx.org

AIDS Services of North Texas (Greenville)
3506 Texas Street
Greenville, TX 75401
(903) 450–4018
http://www.aidsntx.org

AIDS Services of North Texas (Rockwall)
Reeves Service Center
102 S. First Street
Rockwall, TX 75087
(800) 974–2437
http://www.aidsntx.org

Alamo Area Resource Center
527 N. Leona, Bldg. A, Third Floor
P.O. Box 7160
San Antonio, TX 78207
(210) 358–9995
http://www.aarcsa.com

Bryan's House
P.O. Box 35868
Dallas, TX 75235
(214) 559–3946
http://www.bryanshouse.org

Center for AIDS in Houston
P.O. Box 66306
Houston, TX 77266
(713) 527–8219, (888) 341–1788
http://www.centerforaids.org

Montrose Counseling Center
701 Richmond Avenue
Houston, TX 77006
(713) 529–0037
http://www.montrosecounselingcenter.org

Bering Omega Community Services
P.O. Box 540517
Houston, TX 77254
(713) 529–6071
http://beringomega.org

Montrose Clinic
215 Westheimer
Houston, TX 77006
(713) 830–3000
http://www.montroseclinic.org

San Antonio AIDS Foundation
818 E. Grayson
San Antonio, TX 78208
(210) 225–4715
http://www.txsaaf.org

Texas Human Rights Foundation
803 Hawthorne
Houston TX 77006
(800) 828–6417

UTAH

Utah AIDS Information Line
In Utah: (800) 366–2437
National: (801) 487–2100

Utah AIDS Foundation
1408 South 1100 E.
Salt Lake City, UT 84105
(801) 487–2323, (800) 865–5004
http://www.utahaids.org

VERMONT

Vermont AIDS Hotline
In Vermont: (800) 882–2437
National: (802) 863–7245

Chronic Conditions Information Network of Vermont and New Hampshire: HIV/AIDS
P.O. Box 3
Cavendish, VT 05142
(802) 226–7807
http://www.cc-info.net/hiv/hiv_aids.html

Vermont People With AIDS Coalition
P.O. Box 11
Montpelier, VT 05601–0011
(802) 229–5754
http://www.sover.net/~vtpwac

VIRGINIA

Virginia STD/AIDS Hotline
In Virginia: (800) 533–4148
In Virginia Hispanic line: (800) 322–7432
National: (804) 371–7455

AIDS/HIV Services Group Charlottesville
963 Second Street S.E.
Charlottesville, VA 22902
(434) 979-7714, (800) 752-6862
http://www.aidsservices.org

Central Virginia AIDS Resource and Consultation Center
P.O. Box 980147
Richmond, VA 23298
(804) 828-2210, 800-525-7605

Eastern Regional AIDS Resource and Consultation Center
P.O. Box 1980
Norfolk, VA 23501-1980
(757) 446-6170
http://www.evms.edu

AIDS Response Effort
333 West Cork Street, Suite 740
Winchester, VA 22601
(540) 536-5290
http://www.aidsresponseeffort.org

Fredericksburg Area HIV/AIDS Support Services
415 Elm Street
Fredericksburg, VA 22401
(540) 371-7532

Whitman-Walker Clinic of Northern Virginia
5232 Lee Highway
Arlington, VA 22207
(703) 237-4900
http://www.wwc.org/regional_centers/
  nova.html

Williamsburg AIDS Network
P.O. Box 1066
Williamsburg, VA 23187
(757) 220-4606
http://www.williamsburgaidsnetwork.org

WASHINGTON

Washington AIDS Hotline
In Washington: (800) 272-2437
National: (360) 236-3466

BABES Network
1120 E. Terrace, Suite 100
Seattle, WA 98122
(206) 720-5566
http://www.babesnetwork.org

Seattle's Bailey-Boushay House
Bailey-Boushay House
2720 E. Madison
Seattle, WA 98112
(206) 322-5300
http://www.virginiamason.org

Blue Mountain Heart to Heart
2330 Eastgate Street, Suite 105
P.O. Box 40
Walla Walla, WA 99362
(509) 529-4744
Spanish: (509) 529-2174
http://www.bluemountainheart.org

Lifelong AIDS Alliance
1002 East Seneca Street
Seattle, WA 98122
(206) 328-8979
http://www.lifelongaidsalliance.org

Multi-Faith AIDS Project
(206) 324-1520

North American Syringe Exchange Network
535 Dock Street #112
Tacoma, WA 98402
(253) 272-4857
http://www.nasen.org

Pierce County AIDS Foundation
625 Commerce, Suite 10
Tacoma, WA 98402
(253) 383-2565
TTY (253) 627-7830
http://www.piercecountyaids.org

Positive Women's Network
3701 Broadway
Everett, WA 98201
(425) 259-9899, (888) 651-8931
http://www.pwnetwork.org

Seattle AIDS Support Group
(206) 322-2437

Positive Power
(206) 685-4230

Rise N' Shine
417 23rd Avenue S.
Seattle, WA 98144
(206) 628-8949
http://www.risenshine.org

Seattle Shanti
115 16ᵗʰ Avenue
Seattle, WA 98122
(206) 324-1520
http://www.multifaith.org

United Communities AIDS Network
147 Rogers Street N.W.
Olympia, WA 98502
(360) 352-2375
http://www.ucan-wa.org

WEST VIRGINIA

West Virginia AIDS Hotline
In West Virginia: (800) 642-8244
National: (304) 558-2950

AIDS Network
400 West Martin Street
P.O. Box 2306
Martinsburg, WV 25401
(304) 263-0738, (888) 955-6535
http://www.geocities.com/ants25401/

All-Aid International, Inc.
612 Virginia Street E., Suite 202
Charleston, WV 25301
(304) 343-6202

Tri-State AIDS Task Force
821 Fourth Avenue
Huntington, WV 25728
(304) 522-4357

Charleston AIDS Network
P.O. Box 1024
Charleston, WV 25324
(304) 345-4673, (888) 455-4673
http://www.aidsnet.net

Mid-Ohio Valley AIDS Task Force
P.O. Box 1184
Parkersburg, WV 26102
(304) 485-4803

AIDS Task Force of the Upper Ohio Valley
PO Box 6360
Wheeling, WV 26003
(304) 232-6822

WISCONSIN

Wisconsin AIDS Hotline
In Wisconsin: (800) 334-2437
National: (414) 273-2437

AIDS Resource Center of Wisconsin
Appleton Office
130 Washington Street
Appleton, WI 54911
(920) 733-2068, (800) 773-2068
http://www.arcw.org

AIDS Resource Center of Wisconsin
Eau Claire Office
505 Dewey Street S., Suite 107
Eau Claire, WI 54701
(715) 836-7710, (800) 750-2437
http://www.arcw.org

AIDS Resource Center of Wisconsin
Green Bay Office
445 S. Adams Street
Green Bay, WI 54301
(920) 437-7400, (800) 675-9400
http://www.arcw.org

AIDS Resource Center of Wisconsin
Kenosha Office
1212 57th Street
P.O. Box 0173
Kenosha, WI 53141-0173
(262) 657-6644, (800) 924-6601
http://www.arcw.org

AIDS Resource Center of Wisconsin
La Crosse Office
Grandview Center 1702
Main Street, Suite 420
La Crosse, WI 54601
(608) 785-9866, (800) 947-3353
http://www.arcw.org

AIDS Resource Center of Wisconsin
Madison Office
121 S. Pinckney Street, Suite 210
Madison, WI 53701
(608) 258-9103, (800) 518-9910
http://www.arcw.org

AIDS Resource Center of Wisconsin
Milwaukee Office
820 North Plankinton Avenue
P.O. Box 510498
Milwaukee, WI 53203
(414) 273-1991, (800) 359-9272
http://www.arcw.org

AIDS Resource Center of Wisconsin
Superior Office
Board of Trade Building
1507 Tower Avenue, Suite 230
Superior, WI 54880
(715) 394-4009, (877) 242-0282
http://www.arcw.org

AIDS Resource Center of Wisconsin
Schofield (Wausau) Office
1105 Grand Avenue, Suite 1
P.O. Box 26
Schofield, WI 54476
(715) 355-6867, (800) 551-3311
http://www.arcw.org

WYOMING
Wyoming AIDS Hotline
National: (800) 327-3577

PUERTO RICO
**Puerto Rico Linea de Infor SIDA y
Enfermedades de Transmision Sexual**
In Puerto Rico: (800) 981-5721
National: (809) 765-1010

**Puerto Rico Community Network for
Clinical Research on AIDS**
Brimbaugh Street #1162
Urb. Garci'a Ubarri
Rio Piedras
Puerto Rico
(787) 753-9443

Acknowledgments

BY FAR, my editor at Marlowe & Company Renée Sedliar deserves a tip of the hat. She graciously entertained my flights of fancy, but ultimately kept me on target. I've never worked with a better editor. Thank you. Her intern Allison St. John also deserves thanks for an accurate and up-to-date resource guide. Of course, appreciation extends to Marlowe's publisher Matthew Lore for the opportunity to write a second edition of this book and for championing of The First Year series.

In my village, many people deserve recognition: For insights, inspiration, and camaraderie, my friend, coworker, and librarian Katy "ktrino" Mullally. For self-help coaching and puns, Tom Dewan. For years of support and for being a brilliant doctor to us all, Dan Berger. James Haskins for being an equally brilliant therapist and "our group" for *de facto* participation in this book. A nod also goes to Brian Risley and his Hollywood support group.

Everyone on my speed dial earns special mention: Nancy Gottesman for astute lip-pursing and for making my life in LA safe and sane. Diane Baldwin for photography and evolved advice. Mark Heinssen for the majority of his phone calls. Stephanie Gomez for reading, listening, and honesty. Of course, my clan George, Jane, Gail, Lynn, Scott, Bill, Neil, Stefani, and Matthew. Finally, Mike Keeley for love and support since day one.

Index

from lipohypertrophy, 233–34
as long-term side effect, 49
from protease inhibitors, 219
boosted regimens, 87, 142, 218–21
brain health, 23
branched-chain DNA (bDNA) viral load
test, 95, 96, 209–10
BRAT diet, 247
breasts, fat accumulation in, 234
brown fat mitochondria, 232
buffalo hump, 233–34
buprenorphine hydrocholride (Subutex),
149
bupropion (Wellbutrin or Zyban), 137, 141,
224–25
buspirone (BuSpar), 138

Campral (acamprosate calcium), 143
cancer, 119, 120–21, 175, 178
cardio exercise, 179–80
CBC (complete blood count), 68
CD4 cells, 70
CD4+ T-cells. See T-cells
CDC. See Centers for Disease Control and
Prevention
CDC HIV hotline, 44
Celexa (citalopram), 137, 166
Center for HIV/AIDS Educational Studies
and Training, 161
Centers for Disease Control and Prevention
(CDC)
HIV statistics, 5–6
on HIV transmission via anilingus, 107
hotline, 44
on incidence of barebacking, 110–11
on N-9 gel and HIV transmission, 108
name-based reporting rules, 16
study of HIV transmission via oral sex,
106
Centers for Medicare & Medicaid Services,
188
certifications of healthcare professionals,
135
Cervarix, 123
cervical cancer, HPV-related, 119, 120–21
Chantix (varenicline tartrade), 141
children (procreation), 261–65
chimpanzees as origin of HIV, 35
Chinese herbs, 85, 86
chiropractic care, 91
cholesterol
anabolic steroids and, 238–39
blood test for measuring, 48
effect of diet and exercise, 176

heart disease and, 235
HIV and, 177
HIV medications and, 169, 219, 231,
234
chronic hepatitis. See hepatitis B virus;
hepatitis C virus
cirrhosis, 223, 229
citalopram (Celexa), 137, 166
clinical social workers, 135. See also
psychotherapy
clinical trials, 85, 191
clonazepam (Klonopin), 138, 147
COBRA (Consolidated Omnibus Budget
Reconciliation Act of 1985), 188
cocaine, 146–47
cognitive dysfunction
from crystal meth, 152, 153–54, 155
from depression, 129
from efavirenz, 217
low testosterone and, 238
cold sores, 114. See also herpes simplex
virus
Coles, Matthew, 197
colposcopy, 120
combination therapy
for depression, 132
for genital warts, 122
for HIV, 72, 215–16, 218–22
HIV, pregnancy and, 262–63
for overcoming addiction, 141, 149,
157
overview, 72
side effects from, 244–49
trusting your doctor for, 253
comfort foods, 9
community privacy, 15, 17–18
complementary therapies, 85
complete blood count (CBC), 68
compulsion vs. addiction, 162–64
confidentiality, employers,' 203
Consolidated Omnibus Budget
Reconciliation Act of 1985 (COBRA),
188
controlled HIV, 170–71, 173
counselors, 135. See also psychotherapy
coworkers, 55–56, 73–74, 77, 201. See also
workplace
crack cocaine, 146–47
critical threshold for T-cells, 92–93
Crixivan (indinavir), 88–89, 219, 235, 236
crying, 8, 9
cryotherapy, 122
crystal methamphetamine, 151–60
cunnilingus, 106–7, 117–18